CARER'S
HANDBOOK

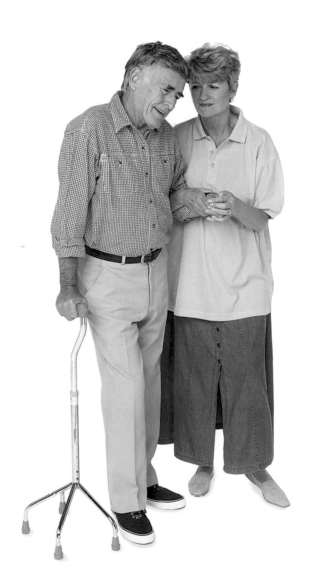

THE VOLUNTARY AID SOCIETIES

St. John Ambulance

St. Andrew's Ambulance Association

British Red Cross

CARER'S HANDBOOK

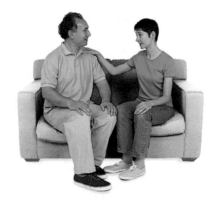

The Authorised Manual of
St. John Ambulance,
St. Andrew's Ambulance Association,
and the British Red Cross

Foreword by HRH The Princess Royal

DORLING KINDERSLEY
LONDON • NEW YORK • SYDNEY • MOSCOW

A DORLING KINDERSLEY BOOK

The St. John Ambulance, a registered charity, St. Andrew's Ambulance Association, a registered charity in Scotland, and the British Red Cross Society, a registered charity, receive a royalty for every copy of this book sold by Dorling Kindersley. Details of the royalties payable to the Societies can be obtained by writing to the Publisher, Dorling Kindersley Limited at 9 Henrietta Street, London WC2E 8PS. For the purposes of the Charities Act 1992 no further seller of the Manual shall be deemed to be a commercial participator with these three Societies.

Managing Editor	Jemima Dunne
Managing Art Editors	Philip Gilderdale and Lynne Brown
Project Editor	Dawn Bates
Editors	Caroline Fraser Ker, Nasim Mawji
Senior Art Editor	Karen Ward
Art Editor	Keith Davis
Designers	Sue Callister, Maria Wheatley
Production	Martin Croshaw
Photography	Andy Crawford

First published in Great Britain in 1997 by
Dorling Kindersley Limited, 9 Henrietta Street, Covent Garden,
London WC2E 8PS

Visit us on the World Wide Web at http://www.dk.com

A CIP catalogue record for this book is available from
the British Library.

ISBN 0-7513-0464-6

Reproduced by Flying Colours SRL, Italy
Printed and bound in Italy by Mondadori, Verona

Publisher's note
The risks associated with lifting and handling tasks covered in this book are complex and each situation must be judged on its own merits. It is unwise to follow the instructions given in this book without proper assessment of the individual circumstances.

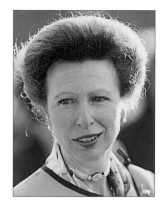

FOREWORD

Many of us, at some time in our lives, will be in the position of caring for someone else. We give care willingly because we love those who are nearest and dearest to us. For some, however, this caring role will become a larger part of their lives taking up more of their time because someone close becomes ill or disabled. Many may find themselves in the position of being a carer.

It is only in recent years that the role of carers has been recognised. Great progress has been made in ensuring that those who work professionally in the care field are aware that carers have needs too and they must be supported in their activities. Carers themselves speak of the need for recognition, respite care and information to help them in their caring role.

It is the need for information which has led to the production of this book which aims to give friendly advice on basic caring skills and pointers on where to go to find further help. It also tries to make clearer the roles of many of the care professionals with whom carers may have contact.

The book has been written by a group of volunteer and paid staff from the three Voluntary Aid Societies, all of whom are experienced carers themselves. It is written not only for carers but for the scores of members from the Societies who voluntarily give support and respite to them.

Everyone needs support and advice when they find themselves in a position of providing care and it is my sincere hope that this book will provide some of that to those who are indeed carers.

Anne

HRH The Princess Royal

CONTENTS

INTRODUCTION

More and more people are being cared for at home, partly because hospitals discharge patients more quickly and also because people live longer. There are around seven million carers in the UK looking after an ill, disabled or elderly person at home. This is the first illustrated and practical guide to address their needs.

BEING A CARER

People become carers for different reasons. You may have chosen to look after a relative at home because he or she has come to depend on you and you do not want him or her to live in a residential home or hospital. Alternatively, you may be a volunteer carer, who has chosen to give up your own time to provide help in the community. Whatever your situation, this book gives you the information you require so that you can provide the best and most rewarding care.

This book outlines – and aims to complement – the support that you can expect from Health and Social Services. We strongly suggest that you make the most of this help and any financial benefits as access to the right information and resources can help you to improve your quality of life and that of the person you are caring for.

THE PERSON YOU ARE CARING FOR

Care needs can vary greatly. Some people may require only a few weeks of help while they recover from an illness or an operation. An elderly, disabled or very ill person, however, may need dedicated care for many months or years. Whoever you are caring for, your aim should be to provide care without depriving the person of his or her independence and dignity.

How This Book Can Help You

This definitive guide to home caring offers practical advice, emotional support and essential information to help you provide the best quality of care possible.

Practical advice Step-by-step photographs show you the best ways to carry out day-to-day tasks, such as giving a bedbath or moving someone safely, with advice on equipment that can help you. A wide range of aids is discussed, such as adapted cutlery, that allow and encourage a physically impaired person to be more independent.

Emotional support The emotional difficulties that both you and your relative may face are addressed and solutions are offered. Case studies are used to highlight – and help you overcome – some of these difficulties. Expert, reassuring advice is offered to guide you through distressing situations.

Essential information There is a comprehensive guide to the resources available to you and your relative, from support groups to financial benefits.

A Guide to the Terms Used	
Gender: throughout the book, we refer to the person being cared for as "he" or "she" alternately from chapter to chapter, except in text that relates directly to an image.	
Relative	The person being cared for. We use this term as most people are related to the person they are caring for. The information in this book, however, is equally relevant if you are caring for a friend or a neighbour.
Home carer	Any person caring for a relative, friend or neighbour in the home environment.
Volunteer carer	Any person working as a carer for a voluntary organisation. There are yellow-tinted pages throughout the book that specifically address the needs of the volunteer carer.
Care/ healthcare professional	A member of the professional care team. The chart overleaf gives details of the professionals and the services that they provide.

CARE PROFESSIONALS

THE CHART BELOW OUTLINES THE PROFESSIONALS with whom you may come into contact while you are caring for your relative. The actual job titles may vary from region to region; the possible alternatives are given in brackets. A care professional who is clinically trained, such as a GP, district nurse or occupational therapist, is known as a "healthcare professional".

CARE PROFESSIONALS AND WHAT THEY DO		
CARE PROFESSIONAL	LOCATION	SERVICES PROVIDED
Social worker (may also be called case worker, care worker or key worker)	Social Services	Assesses the needs of the carer and the person being cared for. Produces a care package and guidance on how to obtain services. Monitors the care provided.
General practitioner (GP)	Health centre/ surgery	A doctor who provides general medical advice and treatment, and can refer patients to a specialist, if necessary.
District nurse (may also be called community nurse)	Health centre/ surgery	Provides general nursing care, such as changing dressings, and assessment of nursing needs. Instructs carers in the use of equipment.
Practice nurse	GP practice/ health centre	Supports the work of the GP, including carrying out a health assessment and advising on diet and lifestyle. Carries out clinical procedures, such as wound dressings and injections.
Health visitor	Health centre/ surgery	Provides health education and advice. Assesses health and social needs of people of all ages.
Community psychiatric nurse/ Community mental health nurse	Health centre or hospital psychiatric unit	Provides support and counselling for those with psychiatric problems; administers medication and monitors overall care and treatment given.
Psychiatric social worker	Social Services or hospital psychiatric unit	Assesses social needs and provides help with practical problems, such as helping a person to fill in an application form for benefits.

CARE PROFESSIONALS AND WHAT THEY DO

CARE PROFESSIONAL	LOCATION	SERVICES PROVIDED
Occupational therapist	Social Services	Assesses a person's individual requirements and advises on adapting the home, equipment and activities to enable him or her to relearn skills and be self-sufficient.
Community physiotherapist	Social Services	Treats those with bone and joint problems. Advises on mobility and exercise.
Speech therapist	Health centre/ hospital	Treats those with speech problems.
Continence adviser	Health centre/ hospital	Provides advice and support, including recommending aids, for those with continence problems.
Stoma care nurse	Health centre/ hospital	Provides advice – on skin care and diet, for example – and support for a person who has a stoma.
Dietician	Hospital	Advises on a healthy diet; tailors special diets to suit specific medical conditions, such as diabetes.
Macmillan nurse	Hospital/hospice	Advises on pain and symptom control for cancer patients. Offers support and counselling for patients and carers.
Marie Curie nurse	Hospital	Provides care for those with cancer. Offers advice and support to the family, including organising short-term care to enable the carer to have a break.
Diabetic liaison nurse	Hospital or GP practice	Advises on the effective control of diabetes, and overall health and welfare matters.
Chiropodist	Hospital/health centre	Offers specialist treatment and therapy for foot problems.
Ambulance personnel	Ambulance station	Provide emergency treatment and transport for patients, and transport to day centres and hospital for day care.

THE VOLUNTARY AID SOCIETIES

THE VOLUNTARY AID SOCIETIES play an essential part in assisting and complementing the work of carers and of Health and Social Services. They provide short- and long-term care at all levels, from helping those recently discharged from hospital to looking after ill, disabled and elderly people.

ST. JOHN AMBULANCE

St. John Ambulance is widely known as the charity that provides comprehensive first-aid training and first-aid assistance at public events. It is committed to providing care and support in the community and its highly valued volunteer schemes help those in need in the community as well as encouraging the personal and social development of many young people. Details of first-aid courses or how to volunteer can be obtained from your local St. John Ambulance office, listed in the telephone directory.

ST. ANDREW'S AMBULANCE ASSOCIATION

St. Andrew's Ambulance Association was founded in 1882, created by the joint efforts of the city's medical profession, business, industry and community interests, as part of a welfare initiative. It is one of Scotland's largest charities, providing training in first aid and allied subjects to over 20,000 people per year. Members of the Association attend 80% of all major sporting and public events and maintain a high level of input into other charitable events in support of, and in aid of, disabled, chronically ill and elderly people.

BRITISH RED CROSS

The British Red Cross was founded in 1870 to care for people in crisis at home and abroad. In the UK its many thousands of volunteers provide a number of essential community services. These include the loan and sale of medical equipment such as wheelchairs, transporting elderly or disabled people who are unable to travel alone and unaided, providing first-aid cover at public events, and helping to care for those recently discharged from hospital. At major emergencies such as floods, evacuations or train crashes, British Red Cross volunteers work alongside the emergency services to give support to those affected, their family and friends.

CHAPTER 1

BEING A CARER

The decision to provide care at home for an ill,
disabled or elderly relative is not one to be taken lightly.
Although caring for someone can be very rewarding, it can also
affect your home and family life, your work and your
free time. If your relative has gradually come to depend on you,
you may have become a carer without realising it.
In this situation, it is still important to decide whether
it is the best option for you. This chapter outlines all aspects of
being a carer, so that you can weigh up the advantages and
disadvantages of looking after your relative at home and
make an informed decision about becoming a
carer or continuing to be one. It may also help you to accept that
caring at home may not necessarily be the best option for you and
your relative. If you do reach this decision, your GP should be able
to advise you on alternative care arrangements.

LOOKING AFTER YOURSELF

To be able to fulfil your role as a carer you
need to maintain your own physical and emotional health.
To achieve this, you need to ask for help and take time off when
you can. This section shows how you can take advantage of the
help that may be on offer – from friends, family, Social Services
and voluntary organisations. Asking for, and accepting, help –
thereby sacrificing less of your own time – can enhance your
relationship with the person that you are caring for.

BECOMING A CARER

Your ROLE AS A CARER, and the length of time it lasts, can vary. If your relative's decline is gradual (as with Alzheimer's disease), caring may be something you are prepared for; but if his decline is sudden (due to a stroke, for example), you may be quite unprepared for looking after him. Whatever the level of care, make sure it is the right choice for both of you.

CASE STUDY

NAME: GRACE
AGE: 67

Grace had been married to Stanley for 45 years. Stanley's health gradually declined and he came to depend more and more on his wife. He began to have minor accidents: a fall left him with a broken arm and he forgot a pan on the cooker, which nearly caused a fire.

Grace did not realise that she had become his carer until she began to fear leaving him alone in the house. Although she wanted to continue to look after him herself, she realised it would be beneficial to both of them if she asked for some help.

Her first step was to look to friends and relatives for help with household chores. Later, a care worker visited and, after a discussion with Grace, arranged for help, which alleviated much of the pressure.

THE LEVEL OF CARE

Your relative may be self-sufficient in many ways, but unable to cope with tasks such as shopping or cleaning; this could mean that he only needs your help for a few hours each week. In more extreme situations, however, you may be looking after someone who requires help with basic needs such as bathing and feeding; in these circumstances, you would be required to provide constant care.

SHORT-TERM CARE

A person recovering from an operation or a major illness will require a high level of care initially. A care plan outlining your relative's needs should be prepared (*see page 33*); if there is any task you think you cannot cope with, you should tell the hospital or your relative's GP. At first, you may be required to help with day-to-day tasks such as cooking or, if your relative has mobility problems, to help him to get from room to room. As he recovers, however, your responsibilities should decrease. Someone who has had a heart attack and is convalescing at home, for example, may require intensive support and care initially, but will gradually regain his strength.

LONG-TERM CARE

If your relative's physical or mental abilities are permanently impaired, you should seriously consider the practicalities of caring for him at home. In most situations quite extensive care needs will have to be considered. Full-time care may be required and may involve adaptations being made to your home – for example, a stairlift may have to be installed, or a downstairs room may have to be converted into a bedroom (*see* Adapting the Home, *pages 43–52*).

IS HOME CARE A PRACTICAL OPTION?

Caring for a relative can be a big responsibility that may affect nearly every aspect of your life. It is essential to have your care situation assessed (*see right*) so that you can consider your own needs and those of your family and relative. Remember, home care is not the only option available to you: if you have doubts, there are other practical alternatives. Before deciding whether to become a carer, or continuing to be one, consider the questions below.

YOU AND YOUR RELATIVE
- Will your relative require long- or short-term care?
- Will he need constant supervision?
- How does he feel about you being his carer?
- Are you the best person to be his carer?
- How much help can you get from friends, family, voluntary agencies and Social Services?
- What other options are available if you don't become the carer?

YOUR PARTNER AND CHILDREN
- How will others in your household be affected?
- Can you fulfil your responsibilities to your relative, as well as to your partner and your children?
- Have you discussed the situation and made the decision as a family?

YOUR HOME
- Will you need to adapt your home?
- If so, will the changes be expensive? Are you eligible for grants (*see page 45*)?

WORK AND FINANCES
- Is it possible to get short-term compassionate leave?
- Are you prepared to give up your job, if necessary?
- Will either of you receive benefits (*see pages 164–68*)?

REASSESSING YOUR DECISION
Your relative's condition may improve or decline over time, affecting his level of dependence on you. Symptoms and circumstances change continually; remember, your first decision need not be final – you can reconsider some of the above factors at a later stage.

GETTING AN ASSESSMENT

As a carer you are entitled to have your needs assessed under the Carers (Recognition and Services) Act 1995 (*see page 172*). The level of help provided can vary from area to area, but do ask what is on offer or you risk losing out.

How you are assessed
An assessor, provided by Social Services, visits your home to talk to you about how you are coping. You will be asked what help you need. Once your requirements have been assessed, a care package may be designed specifically for you, which will take into account the needs and entitlements of you and your relative.

What may be provided
To enable you to take time off (*see page 23*), the package may include help from a sitter or volunteer carer. Your relative may be offered specialist help, such as community nursing, a physiotherapist, a psychiatric social worker or a continence adviser (*see pages 10–11*). You may also be offered help and advice on adapting your home and buying specialist equipment.

BENEFITS OF HOME CARE

ALTHOUGH BEING A CARER is never easy – and there may be times when you will despair – it can be a most rewarding and satisfying experience. There will be demands and challenges to rise to, and you may find that you are forced to draw on previously hidden reserves of strength. Caring can also be a fulfilling experience as you see your relative benefiting from the care provided.

CASE STUDY

NAME: FRANK
AGE: 42

Frank gave up his full-time job to look after his wife, Marjorie, when she became ill with cancer. He and Marjorie had often joked about his culinary skills, which did not stretch beyond boiling an egg. Now, suddenly, he found himself in the position of having to learn how to do everything – look after the children and get them to school on time, cook, do the housework and the shopping – and all on an income that was considerably reduced.

Frank discovered that caring for Marjorie, the children and the home was a full-time job in itself. He also began to understand more about life at home. The experience of caring – and sharing many of the routine tasks – brought the whole family closer together.

BENEFITS FOR YOU

Your role as a carer is ultimately one of giving, but do not forget that there are also benefits for you.

Emotional strength Your relative is likely to rely on you for comfort and support when he is in low spirits and in need of reassurance. You may find that the emotional support you provide strengthens your relationship, bringing you closer together.

Pride You should be able to take pride and satisfaction in the fact that your relative is receiving the best care that you can provide.

Organisational skills Looking after another person requires you to learn to prioritise and organise your time efficiently; these skills can stand you in good stead throughout your life.

BENEFITS FOR YOUR RELATIVE

You are uniquely placed to provide your relative with a quality of life that may not be possible elsewhere.

Independence You can plan your time and structure a typical day together. This will give your relative a level of control and freedom that he may not get in a more ordered environment, such as a residential home.

Personal care The smallest things, from knowing the type of soap your relative prefers, to preparing his favourite meal, can make an immense difference to his quality of life. Maintaining some semblance of normal home life may be very reassuring for him.

Comfort Being cared for at home means that your relative is in familiar surroundings, close to the people and things he knows and loves. He may be reassured to know that you are close at hand to lend emotional support whenever he needs it. He may also want to be close to a pet, such as a dog or cat.

How Relationships Change

CARING FOR SOMEONE can affect your relationship with that person and other people to whom you are close. When someone who was previously fit and healthy becomes dependent because of an illness or disability, power balances shift and roles within a relationship inevitably change. By the same token, some relationships are fortified by the intimacy and closeness that caring brings.

Caring for your Parent

Most of us look up to our parents and rely on them for love and support, even when we have families of our own. It can be very distressing for you when the person you have always relied upon becomes frail or ill, and you may feel that you should assume the responsibility for looking after him. When a parent's health deteriorates, we are all reminded of our mortality. In such situations, role reversal is inevitable but not easy for anyone to accept. It may be difficult for a parent to accept that he is no longer the protector and provider, and must look to you for care. You, on the other hand, may feel you are being pressured into a caring role, and feel guilty for wanting to avoid the responsibility. For many, however, caring for a parent becomes an opportunity to repay them for their help over the years.

Caring for a Child

When a child becomes severely ill or is disabled, the fact that he may have to forego normal development, and may not have the same opportunities as other children, can cause an overwhelming grief. Your instinct will probably be to overprotect your child but, where possible, you should encourage him to learn to do things for himself. Contacting a specialist organisation (*see pages 174–77*) to learn about his illness or disability, and the limitations it will impose, may help you to cope. For example, with the right support, a child with Down's syndrome may develop skills that will enable him to lead a full life. The specialist organisation may also be able to put you in touch with other parents caring for children who have the same illness or disability.

Case Study
Name: John
Age: 27

John discovered that he was HIV-positive and desperately wanted to tell his parents, but dreaded their reaction – his father's in particular. His father had never been able to accept the fact that his son was homosexual and this had been the source of much anger and hostility between them.

When John developed AIDS, his mother insisted that he move home so that she could care for him. This forced them to accept what was happening and to reassess their relationship.

John's return home saw the beginning of a new understanding between him and his parents as they all began to realise that there was no point in punishing each other with recriminations, but that they had to try to accept each other as they were.

THE EFFECTS ON YOUR FAMILY

If your relative comes to live with you, try to involve your partner and your children in his care. This will ease some of the strain on you and will also help your relative to feel that he is part of the household. Your family may be affected in different ways.

Children They may feel neglected, even jealous, especially if you are having to devote more of your time to your relative and less to them. Try to make time for them and, if they want to, involve them in helping you to care for your relative.

Partner Make time for your partner; he too may feel neglected. Try not to take out your frustrations on him, and be as honest and open as possible with each other: hiding your feelings will put an unnecessary strain on your relationship.

Your sex life may be affected: the physical and emotional exhaustion of being a carer can in itself be enough to kill sexual desire. Discuss this with your partner and reassure him that your feelings have not changed.

CARING FOR YOUR PARTNER

Most couples entertain a romantic dream of growing old together. Whether sudden or gradual, the transition of one partner into being a carer brings inevitable change within a relationship: one partner needs to provide more care and support while the other becomes increasingly dependent. It may be a difficult time and you may both have to learn to cope with feelings of sadness: you because the person you love is ill; your partner because he has to adjust to this new, unexpected role of being a dependant.

COPING WITH TASKS

When an illness is physically debilitating, you may have to minister to your partner on quite an intimate level. This may bring you closer together, but you may also find it awkward and embarrassing and want to consider enlisting outside help.

UNDERSTANDING YOUR FEELINGS

If your partner has an illness that affects him mentally, such as Alzheimer's disease, for example, there may be times when you feel that you have lost sight of the person you fell in love with, and become frustrated and angry because you can no longer communicate as you used to. There may even be times when you feel hurt, insulted and angry because your partner becomes confused and does not recognise you. These are natural feelings; if you become exasperated, speak to someone who can understand.

ADAPTING TO A CHANGED SEXUAL RELATIONSHIP

It may be that your partner's illness has changed him physically and that this has affected your sexual relationship. If so, it is important that you share your feelings openly. He may feel ashamed or awkward, and, if he senses that you are becoming distant, it will only reinforce his feelings of isolation. Sex is an important part of a relationship, but people are often shy about discussing it, worrying in silence rather than seeking advice. Sexual desire does ebb, and at times your levels of desire may not be compatible. If you and your partner cannot talk openly, ask your GP to recommend someone who can help.

LOOKING AFTER YOURSELF

A S A CARER, you have responsibilities to yourself as well as to the person you are caring for. Looking after your physical health and being conscientious about your own diet, exercise and sleep will keep you strong and help you to maintain your emotional resilience. If your health begins to suffer, you will not be able to help your relative or yourself.

DIET

If you are busy and your relative has little appetite, you may be tempted to skip proper meals and exist on snacks. Consider the suggestions below as ways of finding time to enjoy a meal:

◆ Regularly invite a friend or relative over for a meal. This will provide a break, as well as some company; it may also inspire you to prepare a meal.

◆ When inviting a friend, or even a group of friends, suggest that everyone contribute a dish to the meal.

EXERCISE

Even though you are physically active as a carer, you should try to make time for regular exercise away from home. This will make you feel more energetic, and provide a break from your daily activities. Try to find the most suitable exercise option.

Exercise classes A class can provide a regular break in your routine; it may also be refreshing to meet people not involved in caring. Can you set aside a block of time each week and be sure that you can keep to it? Could you arrange for a friend to sit with your relative for a couple of hours while you attend a yoga class? Could you go to an exercise class while your relative is at a day centre?

Swimming and walking Timewise, these activities are much more flexible and demand a lower level of commitment than classes. Although more solitary, it may suit you better just to switch off and swim a few lengths of the pool or go for a walk in the park.

Exercising together Is there any way your relative could accompany you to the sports centre? Some local pools run swimming classes for disabled people; this may be a way for you to exercise at the same time.

DO'S & DON'TS

Looking after yourself is an essential part of caring for someone else.

☑ **Do** get enough sleep (*see overleaf*).

☑ **Do** discuss any plans for dieting (with a view to weight loss) with your GP. As a carer, your energy requirements may differ from someone else of your age and build.

☑ **Do** drink plenty of fluids, especially fruit juices.

☑ **Do** eat plenty of fresh fruit and vegetables.

☑ **Do** moderate your alcohol and cigarette consumption.

☒ **Don't** use alcohol or cigarettes as a crutch in stressful moments.

☒ **Don't** snack on cakes and biscuits to maintain energy levels.

☒ **Don't** forego proper, regular meals. This is easy to do, but is not good for you in the long term.

UNDERSTANDING EMOTIONS

CARING CAN BE EMOTIONALLY DRAINING, and you may not always be able to maintain a positive outlook. There may be times when you are confused by your feelings, even ashamed, but the worst thing you can do is to bottle them up. The first step to understanding your feelings is to identify them; it is only then that you can find ways of working them out.

ALLEVIATING TIREDNESS

There is nothing more likely than tiredness and exhaustion to fray your temper and make you irritable. Think about ways in which you can alleviate tiredness.

Planning your day
Draw up a list of your typical daily tasks, then prioritise them. Are they all absolutely necessary? Could you delegate some of them to family or friends? For example, could someone else do the ironing while you have a short rest?

Getting adequate rest
If your relative sleeps in the afternoon, you should try to nap then too. If you have trouble getting to sleep at night, the following tips may help:
◆ try to keep to a regular bedtime routine;
◆ keep the bedroom at a comfortable temperature;
◆ avoid stimulants such as caffeine before bedtime;
◆ don't go to bed hungry.

IDENTIFYING STRESS

It is difficult to avoid becoming stressed; you may often feel that there are not enough hours in the day and that there is no end in sight to the jobs you have to tackle. You may become irritable and moody and feel constantly tired. You may find that on some days even the simplest of tasks, such as the washing up, is just too much to handle. By identifying the signs of stress early on and dealing with them, you can limit their destructive effects.

RECOGNISING AND OVERCOMING STRESS

When you recognise the first signs of stress, try the following stress-reducing tips:
◆ Breathe in deeply and slowly through your nose and out through your mouth. Repeat ten times.
◆ When you are offered time off, use it to spoil yourself. Try not to think about household tasks you could be doing. Get out of the house: visit a favourite place, see a film, have your hair done or visit friends.
◆ If you can't get out, have a long, relaxing bath with essential oils or bath salts. Read a magazine or listen to your favourite music.
◆ Ensure that you go to bed at a reasonable hour, if possible, and that you get enough sleep (*see left*).
◆ Try to take some exercise during the day. If you can't get out of the house, is there an exercise programme on television or video that you can do? Gentle exercise, such as stretching, may be good for both you and your relative, and may be something you can do together; it may even be a source of laughter.
◆ Talk to someone about how you are feeling and, if it helps, have a good cry. A friend, your GP, a specialist organisation or support group (*see pages 174–77*) may be able to listen and help.

UNDERSTANDING ANGER AND GUILT

It is only human to feel angry when something happens that hurts you or upsets your plans. This is a natural and healthy response, especially when someone you love falls ill or becomes disabled. Anger is a complex emotion, often suppressed because we feel guilty about expressing it. If you can get to the root of your anger, you will have gone part of the way towards dealing with it, and also with the accompanying guilt. There are certainly times when anger needs to be controlled, but it should never be ignored. Here are some of the more common reasons why you, as a carer, may experience anger and guilt:

♦ someone you love is suffering;

♦ the illness or disability has upset all your future plans together, and you feel guilty about feeling angry;

♦ you feel angry with your relative for being ill and, even though you know this is irrational, it does not stop you feeling this way;

♦ you feel that the situation is unjust, that neither you nor your relative deserves what is happening;

♦ it may be an expression of the frustration you feel as a carer; you may simply feel that you cannot cope.

CASE STUDY

NAME: HARRY   AGE: 72

Harry, who cared for his wife Margaret – a sufferer of Parkinson's disease – began to feel increasingly angry and isolated. The family GP suggested that he contact a carers' support group so that he could talk to others in similar situations.

Harry confessed to a carer who visited him that he sometimes felt angry because Margaret could no longer do the things she had once been able to, and sometimes did not even recognise him. He felt angry because his wife was slow and uncommunicative, then he felt guilty because he knew she could not help it. The carer visiting told him that she, too, had felt anger, and also the grief that came with seeing someone you love deteriorate.

Harry now relies on the group for support; he knows that there are other carers he can talk to who will understand his frustration about doing everything he can for Margaret, but still feeling it is never quite enough.

DO'S AND DON'TS

Anger can get out of control and lead to irrational judgements and decisions, even violence.

☑ **Do** discuss your problems with the GP or care professional; either may be able to refer you to someone who can help.

☑ **Do** seek the help of a specialist organisation (*see pages 174–77*) that has knowledge of your relative's illness; they will be able to empathise with your situation and offer you and your relative advice and support.

☑ **Do** get away from your relative for a few minutes if you feel yourself becoming tense. First, make sure he can be safely left on his own.

☑ **Do** try to understand that your relative may feel angry and frustrated at times. He may also feel guilty about having to rely on you so much.

☒ **Don't** cut yourself off from friends because you are angry with them for not sharing your suffering. You will only isolate yourself further and become embittered.

☒ **Don't** be ashamed of your anger. Talk about your feelings before they become overwhelming.

SEEKING COUNSELLING

Carers often face problems that seem insurmountable.

Can counselling help?
Counselling is one way of helping people adjust and come to terms with their difficulties; it is also good for exploring practical ways to solve problems. Counselling is not a "cure" for people with psychiatric or physical illnesses and it is not psychotherapy, which is a treatment for people with specific mental health problems.

Choosing a counsellor
The availability of counselling varies widely across the country, and choosing a counsellor can be difficult. Some private counsellors advertise their services, others are linked to voluntary organisations. The British Association for Counselling (*see page 177*) can supply a list of registered private counsellors in your area. Increasingly, counsellors are attached to GP surgeries and available on the National Health Service. Your GP should also be able to assess your needs to see if specialist treatment, such as psychotherapy, is required.

COPING WITH LONELINESS AND ISOLATION

It is easy to become isolated as a carer. You may find that you are too busy to keep up with friends and relatives. If people visit less frequently, it may be because they see that you are busy, and worry that they may be in the way. Sometimes people stop visiting because they are embarrassed about your relative's illness. The following positive steps may help:
◆ make time to contact people and reassure them that you still need their friendship and support;
◆ try to be open and honest about your feelings and your needs – don't shut people out or try to pretend that you can cope on your own. To feel happy in your caring role you also need to feel supported and loved;
◆ be open about your relative's illness and what it means in terms of daily care;
◆ offer reassurance to people if they are frightened or upset by the signs of the illness – remember that they are not as familiar as you are with the situation;
◆ enlist the help of friends and relatives, and involve them in the care if you can. People are often happier if they know they are making a positive contribution.

RECOGNISING DEPRESSION

There may well be times when everything gets on top of you, when you don't know where you will find the resolve to go on. Normally these feelings will pass if you talk to a friend, get a good night's sleep or take a break. Sometimes, however, they persist and develop into depression, which can be destructive. Some of the more common symptoms of depression to watch out for are:
◆ tearfulness;
◆ irritability;
◆ tiredness;
◆ feelings of inadequacy;
◆ lack of concentration;
◆ fitful sleep, or too much sleep;
◆ eating all the time, or complete loss of appetite.
If you are experiencing any of these symptoms and you feel that you can't discuss your feelings with a friend, you might want to consider seeking impartial advice from a counsellor or GP (*see left*).

FINDING TIME FOR YOURSELF

LOOKING AFTER SOMEONE FULL-TIME is a demanding job. At times you will need a break, not only from daily chores, but also from your relative, for either a few hours, a day, a week or longer. To do this you will need respite care. Respite care ranges from someone sitting with your relative for an afternoon or your relative going into a residential home for a short stay.

MAKING TIME FOR YOURSELF

You may feel guilty about wanting to have a break, feeling that it implies that you do not care about your relative. However, there are many reasons why it is *essential* to take time away from caring.

To reduce stress levels Being stressed will mean that you are more prone to illness, irritability and depression. Carers often soldier on unaided, denying themselves any relief until their own health suffers. Time away can help you to put things in perspective.

To improve your caring relationship To keep a relationship alive and interesting, you need to talk to other people and have other experiences. The relationship that you have with your relative is no different: time apart will almost certainly give both of you new perspectives and different things to talk about.

For your independence Your relative is necessarily dependent on you, the carer, but remember that you also need care, not least in the form of emotional support. Spend time keeping up with friends and family and maintaining your own social life. Try to carry on with a hobby, if you have one. Retaining some degree of independence will mean that you are less likely to become isolated and feel overwhelmed.

ARRANGING RESPITE CARE

You can arrange a short break yourself (for example, by asking a friend to care for your relative for the afternoon), but help can also be provided by social services, your local health authority or trust, and voluntary associations. The care provided, and who provides it, will depend upon the severity of your relative's condition. You might also consider a care attendant scheme, which provides care in the home. For respite care options, see the chart overleaf.

RESIDENTIAL RESPITE CARE

If you are thinking of taking a break for a week or more, one option is for your relative to go to stay in a residential care home. Consider the following when you are choosing a temporary care home:

- Is it registered with the local authority?
- Are the staff experienced in dealing with your relative's particular needs?
- Does your relative like the place?
- Is it well-kept and clean?
- What is the food like?
- Are the staff friendly?
- Are temporary residents fully integrated into the life of the home? Can they participate in outings?
- Are there others having a temporary break?
- Is it tastefully decorated and comfortably furnished?

RESPITE CARE

THE BEST TYPE OF RESPITE CARE for your relative will depend on his particular requirements, the length of time you will be away and the cost involved. Cost and availability will vary according to the area in which you live. If you require only a short break, it may be worth asking family and friends for help in caring for your relative.

TYPE OF CARE	LENGTH OF BREAK	SERVICES PROVIDED
Day centre	A day or more a week, as required.	This will vary from centre to centre, but may include occupational therapy such as art, amateur dramatics, keep fit and craft work. Services such as hairdressing may also be available.
Hospital	As required.	Complete medical and nursing care, including rehabilitation. Some hospitals offer spiritual support.
Hospice	According to requirements, it could be from days to weeks.	Pain and symptom relief, spiritual support, counselling service, clergy and alternative therapies, such as massage. Home sitting service may be available.
Residential care home/Nursing home	1–2 weeks.	This will vary from home to home, but may include occupational therapy such as art, amateur dramatics, keep fit and craft work. Services such as chiropody may also be available.
Sitting service	Day or night, as arranged.	Day or night nursing, general care and supervision.
Voluntary help	A few hours/daily.	Outings or home help.
Private nurse	Depends on means and requirements.	Any nursing care appropriate to your relative's requirements, from changing dressings and giving injections to giving a bath.
Holiday	1–2 weeks.	Varies, depending on whether it is a purpose-built holiday centre or a hospital with flats.

How Can Family and Friends Help?

Some people will be keen to help but may be unsure as to exactly how. Here are some suggestions:

◆ Could someone sit with your relative for a few hours to give you a chance to rest or go out?

◆ Could a member of the family come and stay occasionally, or could your relative go and stay with him or her?

◆ Could someone help with the ironing, hoovering, laundry or washing up?

◆ Could anyone help with small tasks such as shopping or picking up a prescription?

Level of Care	Where to Find out What is Available
From attendant to registered nurse, but it depends on staffing levels and whether or not people who have certain conditions are catered for.	Social services, health authority, voluntary organisations, library, local press and GP's surgery; health board in Scotland. Referral from your relative's GP.
Doctors and registered nurses. Social services coordinator. Specialist help, such as physiotherapy.	Referral from your relative's GP.
Full care with specialist doctors, registered nurses and complementary medicine specialists.	Social services, referral from your relative's GP, community nursing, local paper, library. Admittance normally limited to those with cancer or those who are terminally ill.
Residential care home: usually care assistants with additional medical cover by GPs and district nurses. Nursing home: the above and registered nurses.	Social services, referral from your relative's GP, local paper, library, support groups, voluntary organisations. Social services in some areas may help with fees.
Volunteers or registered nurses.	Social services, voluntary organisations, support groups, hospices, community nursing services.
May not be specialised. Depends on your relative's requirements.	Neighbour, friends, family, support groups, voluntary organisations.
Registered nurse.	Nursing agency, GP. Cost may be a limitation as private nurses can be expensive.
Your relative can go by himself or you can both go together (see overleaf). Trained staff may be on hand to assist.	Holiday organisations (see page 174). Grants may be available from some organisations, and some, such as Arthritis Care (see page 174), have their own holiday homes.

GOING ON HOLIDAY TOGETHER

Caring for your relative does not mean that you have to be permanently confined to the home. Respite holidays enable your relative to have a holiday – in the care of someone else – thereby also affording you a break. If you want to go on holiday together, there are several organisations that arrange holidays for those with special care needs. There may also be grants available.

FACILITIES CHECKLIST

Before booking a holiday, check that the facilities are suitable for your relative's needs:
◆ Is there wheelchair access to all areas – to the dining room, gardens and lifts, for example?
◆ Is the accommodation accessible to someone with limited mobility? Is your relative's room on the ground floor, for example?
◆ Is there a lift/stairlift?
◆ Are there facilities for disabled people, such as handrails in the toilet, bathroom and shower?
◆ Are there bed and bath hoists?
◆ Are there bed lifts/ different bed heights?
◆ Are there facilities for guide dogs?
◆ Are registered nurses, care assistants or trained medical staff available?
◆ Are treatments, such as physiotherapy or hydrotherapy available?

CHOOSING A HOLIDAY

Holidays that cater specifically for the needs of ill or disabled people are available: these provide different levels of care depending on individual needs.

PLANNING AHEAD
Make sure you discuss any special needs and the level of care required with the tour operator beforehand (*see left*). Most can offer useful information, such as the location of purpose-built holiday centres and whether or not there are carers on hand to assist with daily care, such as helping someone to eat.

CONTACTING SPECIALIST ORGANISATIONS
In the UK, contact the Holiday Care Service (*see page 174*), a charity that provides information about low-cost holidays with accommodation and transport facilities for ill or disabled people. The aim of the service is to give carers and their relatives the confidence to travel away from home. To ensure an up-to-date database of the level and standard of care on offer, the charity works closely with holiday and tour operators. For example, you can find out which holiday centres have trained staff available to give medication or help with washing and dressing. The British Red Cross (*see page 174*) also arranges large annual holidays for disabled people.

GETTING THERE
A local voluntary aid organisation may be able to assist with travel arrangements, such as transport to and from stations and airports, or the travel company itself may be able to organise this. Most rail companies offer help, and airlines are obliged to give "on and off" assistance, and help at airports, to people who have mobility problems.

SUPPORT GROUPS

PEOPLE WHO SHARE EXPERIENCES of a particular type of illness or disability often form groups so that they can offer support and understanding to each other, and share tips on how to cope. There are two types of support group: those formed to provide information about a particular condition, offering help to you and your relative, and those that are there to support the carer.

WHY JOIN A SUPPORT GROUP?

By joining a support group you can benefit from meeting new people in a similar situation to yourself and offer and receive help and advice.

To meet others in a similar situation The life of a carer can be a very isolated one: meeting and sharing your experiences with others in the same position can be life-affirming in itself.

To have a break It is understandable to want time away from your caring role. Support groups will often find someone to sit with your relative, and may be able to arrange transport to and from the meeting.

To obtain information Often, particularly if an illness is rare, and experience in dealing with the symptoms is limited, support groups can provide an opportunity for carers and their relatives to meet and pool their knowledge. These groups often offer specialist training as well. Support groups can also keep you up-to-date regarding benefits and your rights as a carer.

For support Members of the groups are usually carers, ex-carers or sufferers themselves, so are well placed to understand your problems and offer practical advice and support. Because they are or have been in your position, they will be able to identify with your feelings and reassure you that you are not alone.

FINDING THE RIGHT SUPPORT GROUP

Many support groups are formed specifically for people coping with or caring for someone with a particular disease or disability. There are also many more general groups; in the UK, for example, the Carers National Association campaigns on issues such as benefits, recognition and support for all carers. They have a head office and a network of local groups nationwide (*see page 174*).

FORMING A SUPPORT GROUP

If you cannot find a suitable group, consider starting one yourself: the Carers National Association provides a free information pack.

Get others interested Advertise locally for others with similar experiences to contact you. The GP or district nurse may be able to help you start up a group.

Arrange a meeting Fix a date, a time and a suitable venue, for example, a GP's surgery or village hall.

Clarify your aims Is there a particular cause you wish to champion or do you just want to meet people in the same position as yourself?

Confidentiality Agree on confidentiality from the start. No one will feel relaxed if they fear that their experiences may be discussed outside the group.

ARE YOU COPING?

IT IS POSSIBLE THAT YOU AND YOUR RELATIVE may find that home care is not practical. While many adapt easily to the role of home carer, some, understandably, find it difficult to cope. Bear in mind, too, that circumstances may have changed and it may be time to look at alternatives for care. It is important, however, that you are both happy with the final decision.

PINPOINTING PROBLEMS

It may help to draw up a rough schedule detailing your daily care duties, then pinpoint areas where you need help. You can then use this information to get a perspective on a typical week. An early morning routine might look something like this:

◆ 7am Get up – wash and have breakfast;

◆ 7.30 Get Anna up, give breakfast;

◆ 8.30 Help Anna into shower and assist with washing her;

◆ 9.15 Dress Anna;

◆ 9.30 Dress myself then do some housework.

Do you need help in the mornings? Has it become too much of a physical strain to move your relative, for example? Seek advice from a care professional who may be able to help you assess the situation and find alternative ways of meeting your care needs.

ASSESSING YOUR SITUATION

To find out if home care is still a practical option for you, examine your day-to-day routine and consider how you are feeling physically and emotionally.

Organisation Is there a routine to your day? Are you managing your time as efficiently as possible?

Priorities Are you wasting time and energy on unnecessary tasks and problems that will only increase your stress levels?

Support Are you getting all the help you can? Have you considered all your options: friends, relatives, voluntary organisations and social services?

Financial entitlements Are you claiming the benefits to which you are rightfully entitled (*see pages 164–68*)?

Physical health Are you eating and sleeping properly? Are you able to exercise on a fairly regular basis?

Emotional health Are you able to maintain a rational outlook? Do you feel on top of things at most times? If not, do you have a friend or a counsellor with whom you can share your feelings?

Breaks Are you getting enough time for yourself? Are you taking regular weekly breaks or holidays?

Independence Can you get out to see friends? Do you still have a social life?

Commitments Can you keep commitments to others in your family and to yourself?

A PERSPECTIVE ON YOUR DECISION

If at any stage you decide that you can no longer care for your relative at home, do not feel guilty or think that you have failed. It will probably be in the best interests for both of you if he is provided with alternative care, especially if he needs more specialised help and supervision than you are able to provide.

CHAPTER 2

BEING A VOLUNTEER CARER

A volunteer may be required to look after a
person if there is no friend or relative to act as a carer.
A volunteer may also be required to help a home carer; either to
allow him to take time off or to help him with strenuous tasks
that he cannot carry out alone, such as helping his
relative to get out of bed or into the bath.
Health and Social Services increasingly rely on voluntary
organisations and the volunteer carers who work for them, to
provide both short- and long-term support.

THE ROLE OF THE VOLUNTEER

As a volunteer, you may be supervised and
supported by a care professional, such as a district nurse, who is
responsible for prescribing and reviewing the needs of the person
and who will advise you on the level of care that is required.
Integral to your role is the ability to get on with people – the
person being cared for, the home carer, if there is one, and the
professionals with whom you may work. In order to provide the
best service, you should feel fulfilled in your role, which means
being able to address problems and ask for help when necessary.
Being a volunteer can be hard work and is sometimes very
challenging, but ultimately it can be a highly
rewarding and satisfying experience.

BECOMING A VOLUNTEER

PEOPLE OF ALL AGES can volunteer to become carers: voluntary organisations welcome the help of anyone who is willing to give up time to assist others. To make enquiries, telephone or write to your local library to request information about the type of voluntary care taking place in your community, and advice on how you can get involved.

WHAT DOES IT INVOLVE?

Becoming a volunteer carer may be a daunting prospect for many people. Below are some of the most common questions asked by potential volunteers.

WILL I BE INTERVIEWED?

You will probably be interviewed and asked for references; you may be required to sign a form declaring that you do not have any health problems or a criminal record. You may also meet other volunteers in your area, who will explain the procedure for becoming a carer and what the work involves.

WHAT KIND OF WORK IS INVOLVED?

The type of work can vary from a couple of hours a day spent helping an elderly person with gardening, to sitting overnight with someone who is ill. You will never be expected to be involved in any task, or care for any person, if it makes you feel uncomfortable.

WHAT SKILLS DO I NEED?

You do not need any specialist skills to volunteer to be a carer. You will, however, be offered training ranging from how to communicate with a wide variety of people, to basic first-aid and care skills. The skills gained as a volunteer will help you in all walks of life, and working in the community is widely respected by employers. The experience you gain may be accredited to other training schemes.

HOW MANY HOURS WILL I HAVE TO WORK?

The number of hours you agree to work is entirely up to you; you can arrange times to suit your lifestyle and other commitments. You can be flexible, but you must give notice if you cannot carry out your duties.

WORKING WITH PROFESSIONALS

YOU MAY BE REQUIRED to liaise with a number of professional people, such as community nurses and social workers. These people are responsible for assessing the level of care needed by the person you are caring for, and ensuring that it is carried out. When working with care professionals, you will be under their guidance, complementing, rather than replacing, their duties.

UNDERSTANDING YOUR ROLE

The care professional will delegate tasks to you or ask you to assist him. You may also be required to help a home carer so that he is able to have some time off.

BEING RELIABLE

Reliability is a key element in your relations with professional care workers. If you cannot meet a commitment, you should always try to give plenty of notice so that alternative arrangements can be made. If you cancel at the last minute, or fail to turn up at all, you will be letting down the person being cared for and may be compromising the good name of the voluntary organisation for which you work.

FOLLOWING A CARE PLAN

Health and Social Services may give you a care plan (*see page 33*) that has been devised following an assessment of the person requiring care. If you are given such a plan, you should always adhere to the recommendations made in it.

The type of care The requirements of the person being cared for and the kind of activities you will need to carry out.

The level of care The extent and frequency of the care you will give to that person.

The objectives of the care What specific aims the care plan is trying to achieve.

WHAT YOU CAN OFFER

You may see the person you are caring for more often than the care professional. If you notice improvements or a deterioration in the person's health, or recognise any deficiencies in the care plan, you should mention these and suggest possible changes.

CASE STUDY

NAME: EMMA
AGE: 32

Emma began caring for Mr Thomas, who was confined to bed for most of the time because of a serious back injury. On her first visit, she referred to the care plan she had been given by the district nurse. This stated that Mr Thomas would require a bed bath, which Emma had been trained to do.

After caring regularly for Mr Thomas for a month, his condition improved. Based on past experience, and after discussing it with him, Emma felt that he might now be fit enough to get into a bath by himself.

Emma knew it was not within the scope of her duties to change the care orders. However, she suggested the change to the district nurse, who reassessed Mr Thomas's condition during her next visit and altered the care orders accordingly.

CARING FOR SOMEONE

EVEN THOUGH, AS A VOLUNTEER CARER, you are not a qualified professional, you should not think of yourself as an amateur. It is important that you act professionally so that the person you are caring for trusts you. Although you may become a close companion or a friend, you should still remember to behave responsibly and maintain confidentiality at all times.

THE HOME CARER

As a volunteer carer, you may be in close contact with a home carer. Your relationship with that person is as important as your relationship with the person being cared for. It is essential that you work well as a team.

Practical support You can help with day-to-day tasks or provide night-time care so that the home carer has some time to himself. You can also make sure that he has been offered and, if he wants to, is making use of all the resources that are available to him. For example, he may welcome your help in obtaining advice and information about the financial benefits to which he may be entitled.

Emotional support The home carer may lead an isolated life, and may find the burden of caring very arduous. Just being there to support and listen to him may help.

SATISFY THE NEEDS OF THE CARED FOR

The most important aspect of your voluntary role is to provide care without depriving the person of her independence and self-confidence.

Individuality The person being cared for has needs and preferences that should be respected. Try to understand why she may be acting in a certain way.

Independence Wherever possible, allow the person to make decisions and do things for herself, even if this means that a task takes longer. Always ask her opinion and respect her views.

Confidence If the person being cared for feels she is a burden to everyone, she will become lonely and insecure. Comfort and reassure her, and encourage her to focus on the skills and abilities she still has.

BE AWARE OF YOUR OWN LIMITATIONS

As a volunteer you will be giving much of your time to others, and may be dealing with stressful situations. If you are dissatisfied or unhappy, it will be difficult for you to provide the best care.

Having limited skills You may feel that you have not been fully trained or are not qualified to deal with some of the tasks required of you, and that you are encroaching on the work of the care professional.

Feeling uncomfortable It may be that you don't get on with the person you are caring for, or feel ill at ease in the environment in which you are working.

Being unable to give enough You may feel that you are being asked to provide more care than you are able to offer.

Try to recognise your own limitations and, if they affect the quality of the care you are providing, discuss them with your supervisor.

How a Care Plan can Help you

When someone needs care, a plan is essential as it provides a clear breakdown of the person's requirements. It can be used by other volunteer carers or care professionals who come into the home. The plan should be provided by a care professional, who may ask you to help devise it or make recommendations. If, for any reason, it is not provided, request one from your supervisor or seek specific guidance about the type of care that the person requires. An example of a care plan is shown below.

CARE PLAN	NAME: BETTY FRASER AGE: 91
ACTIVITY	**ASSESSMENT**
Mobility	Mobile with the use of a walking stick. A wheelchair should be used for long distances.
Washing	Can wash unaided; needs help to get into and out of the bath.
Dressing	Needs basic supervision.
Eating	Needs some help and encouragement. Prefers to eat with a spoon from a bowl, so cut food up or give soft foods if possible. Likes hot chocolate in the evening.
Continence	No problem.
Sight	Poor vision, even with spectacles.
Hearing	Adequate. Good with the use of an aid.
Behaviour	Mildly confused at times. Should be informed about any visitors.
Medication	Twice daily for arthritis, with morning and evening meals.
Communication	Mostly retains information and indicates needs verbally.
Finances	Managed by her daughter.
Social activities	Enjoys joining arranged activities. Attends day centre alternate weeks on a Wednesday.
Hobbies	Enjoys listening to the radio and having the newspaper read to her.
Level of care	Betty needs care twice daily from Monday to Friday (her daughter cares for her at weekends). She should be visited first thing in the morning and in the afternoon. She receives Meals on Wheels at lunchtime, but her evening meal should be prepared for her.
Objectives of care	Betty is quite able, and should be encouraged to be independent. Regular attendance at a day centre has been successful. Aim for attendance at least once a week by the end of the year.

SIGNS OF ABUSE

Evidence suggests that abuse is more likely to be the result of poor pre-existing relationships, or alcohol or mental health problems, rather than due to the strain of caring. However, abuse does occur and it could be the carer or the cared for who is the abuser. If you suspect abuse of any kind, inform your supervisor who will deal with it through the correct channels. Do not share your suspicions with anyone else.

Physical abuse Look out for physical signs such as negative body language (*see page 38*) and bruising.

Emotional abuse This might be one person shouting constantly at the other, belittling her or keeping her isolated. It may result in the victim of abuse being quiet and withdrawn.

Financial abuse If you notice any financial irregularities, or stealing from the person you are caring for, inform your supervisor. Keep receipts for goods that you buy on behalf of the person, so that your conduct is beyond reproach.

HOW TO TREAT THE CARED FOR

The way you treat the person you are caring for will affect how she feels about herself. It is important that you respect her needs and that she trusts you. If respect and trust are established early on, you should be able to form a mutually beneficial relationship.

RESPECT THE INDIVIDUAL

When caring for someone, treat her with the utmost respect. Ask yourself, "How would I like to be treated?", and make this the basis for the standard of care that you want to achieve. Find out as much as you can about the person you are caring for, and respect her individual needs. She may, for example, have specific dietary needs (*see page 64*), be of a different sexual orientation or different culture (*see page 37*). Never forget that the person you are caring for is an individual in her own right, and is entitled to know what is happening to her. If there are changes to the care orders, take the time to explain them to her and, if possible, involve her in any decisions.

MAINTAIN CONFIDENTIALITY

It is important that the person you are caring for trusts you. To achieve this trust, you should respect her privacy and maintain confidentiality at all times. You have a duty to keep any information you may learn in your caring role absolutely confidential, including anything contained in the person's care records. The only exception to this is if you suspect abuse of any kind (*see left*); report this to your supervisor immediately, but do not talk about it to anyone else.

ADDRESSING PROBLEMS

You may not immediately feel at ease with the person you are caring for, but, over time, you may be able to develop a good relationship. In some circumstances, however, you may be completely incompatible with the person, to the point where you cannot carry out care duties effectively. If these differences cannot be resolved, ask to be removed from the duties. Remember, however, to strive for professionalism, even when you cannot communicate effectively with the person you are caring for.

CHAPTER 3

COMMUNICATION

Talking and listening to one another are essential
human needs. People need to communicate in order to express
their anxieties and emotions, and to make their wishes known.
Keeping the communication channels open when caring for
your relative can be beneficial to both of you, and it is important
to know what to do when this becomes difficult.

COMMUNICATION SKILLS

Most human beings take verbal communication
for granted, so much so that they may, sometimes, not
bother to make time for conversation. When you are caring for
your relative, making the time to talk and listen can enhance
your relationship and help to iron out any difficulties.
You may be caring for someone with impaired
senses, for whom verbal communication may be impossible; in
such a situation you may need to rely on non-verbal skills, such as
reading his body language and thinking about
how you use your own. Do not, for example, be
afraid to use touch, which can be reassuring as well as being
an effective way of conveying your feelings. You will also
need to explore ways to help your relative to
improve his communication skills. This may be achieved by
seeking specialist help and finding
out if there are any aids available that cater
for your relative's particular needs.

TALKING AND LISTENING

FINDING TIME FOR CONVERSATION is very important, especially to someone who is housebound or does not have contact with many people. It is easy to find excuses not to talk or listen, but if you make the time you may feel closer to the person you are caring for. Proper communication will allow both of you to express your feelings and help to prevent resentment building up.

DO'S & DON'TS

☑ **Do** try to think about the way you are speaking and how your voice sounds. The pitch, rate and rhythm of your voice are important if your relative has impaired hearing (*see page 41*).

☑ **Do** be patient if your relative has impaired speech (*see page 39*). Give him time to finish his sentence and resist the temptation to interrupt or speak for him.

☒ **Don't** patronise your relative. Whatever his disability, he should be treated with respect and not be addressed as if he were a child. A person who is physically impaired is still likely to be mentally alert.

☒ **Don't** exclude your relative from group conversations, whatever his condition. It may make him feel isolated and worthless if he is left alone in a corner watching and listening to other people talking.

IMPROVING COMMUNICATION

There are many reasons why communication can break down, making it difficult for you and your relative to talk to each other. It is important to keep the lines of communication open and address any problems as early as possible.

MAKE TIME TO TALK

If you and your relative spend long periods of time together, you may become so familiar with each other that you do not notice hours passing without conversation. Also, as a carer, you will undoubtedly be extremely busy, and it may seem like a luxury to sit down and talk. But try not to think of it like that; allocate time to talk, even if it is only over a cup of tea or between television programmes. It could mean a lot to your relative.

FIND COMMON INTERESTS

If your own lifestyle is restricted, it may be difficult to find things to talk about. However, it is usually possible to find subjects of mutual interest, such as sport, gardening or television. Do not be afraid to talk about yourself and your interests. If your friends visit, try to include your relative in the discussions.

BE PATIENT

If your relative suffers from confusion or has impaired speech or hearing, verbal communication can be difficult and frustrating. You may sometimes feel that your patience is being pushed to the limit. Instead of getting angry, try taking deep breaths to calm yourself down or, after ensuring that your relative is safe, leave the room for a few minutes until you are feeling less wound up.

Being a Volunteer Carer

W HEN YOU ARE A CARER from outside the home, it is essential to communicate effectively with the person you are looking after and the home carer, if there is one. This may range from the simple matter of addressing someone appropriately, to overcoming language or cultural differences. Finding out as much as possible about the person you are caring for will help.

Language and Cultural Differences

If the person you are caring for speaks a different language, communication can be difficult, but over time it should become easier. Be aware of any different cultural beliefs, and respect the fact that he may want to do things in a different way.

Use an interpreter
You may find that younger members of the family speak fluent English. Communicate either through one of them or ask your supervisor to arrange for an interpreter to accompany you, at least initially.

Obtain bilingual material
You can obtain information about relevant bilingual material, such as books and leaflets, from your local authority or the Health Education Authority.

Educate yourself
Find out as much as possible about the person's beliefs by speaking to him or his family, and by obtaining information from your supervisor or local authority.

Respect the person's wishes
Beliefs and traditions may affect someone's lifestyle; this could include dietary restrictions (*see page 65*) or a woman not being allowed to be seen by a male doctor.

Be aware of isolation
Some members of ethnic minorities may have no contacts outside their immediate family, which may lead to a feeling of isolation. Discuss this problem with the affected person and his family, and try to find local activities that enable him to meet people who share his beliefs and interests.

Relating to the Home Carer

If there is already a carer in the home, she may resent your presence or even see it as an intrusion. Reassure her that you are there to support her and not to take over. Work with her to identify ways in which you can help.

Advice and support
You may be able to help with practical problems and, if she asks for it, give advice on the benefits and resources that are available to her.

Companionship The home carer may not come into contact with many people; she may welcome a friendly face and the chance to talk to someone else.

Level of care If you and the home carer communicate well with each other and work together, the overall level of care given should improve, which will be beneficial to the person being cared for.

USING BODY LANGUAGE

ALTHOUGH MOST OF US express ourselves through the spoken word, we also communicate in many non-verbal ways. When you are caring for your relative, it can help if you understand his body language and know how to use your own. Body language is even more important if your relative's speech and hearing are impaired, rendering him unable to communicate verbally.

SIGNS OF ABUSE

You may suspect from your relative's body language that he is the victim of physical or emotional abuse. Abuse can take place in the home, as well as when the person is being cared for elsewhere. If you suspect abuse of any kind (*see page 34*), alert a care professional, but do not tell anyone else of your suspicions. Look out for behavioural changes or signs of injury.

Withdrawal The abused may isolate himself. He may appear wary of people and withdraw when he is approached.

Depression He may appear depressed or unusually quiet and avoid communication, especially eye contact.

Injury The abused may try to cover up bruising or other injuries. He may give unlikely explanations for how he has sustained his injuries.

THE PERSON BEING CARED FOR

Learning to read body language will help you to care more effectively for your relative.

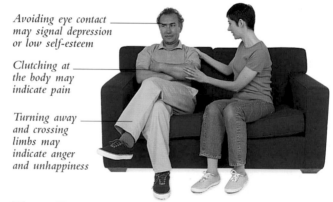

Avoiding eye contact may signal depression or low self-esteem

Clutching at the body may indicate pain

Turning away and crossing limbs may indicate anger and unhappiness

THE CARER

You can use your body language to help your relative feel more secure and so improve communication.

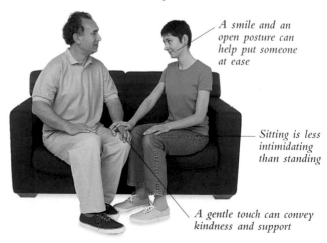

A smile and an open posture can help put someone at ease

Sitting is less intimidating than standing

A gentle touch can convey kindness and support

ADAPTING FOR SPECIAL NEEDS

COMMUNICATION DIFFICULTIES may arise when you are caring for someone with impaired speech, sight or hearing. It is possible to overcome these difficulties by adapting the way in which you communicate. Many aids are available to help someone who has impaired senses to improve his ability to communicate and encourage independence.

IMPAIRED SPEECH

Helping someone to relearn how to speak can take a long time, and requires a great deal of perseverance, patience and encouragement. Talk to your relative's GP to find out what specialist help is available.

REASONS FOR SPEECH LOSS

There are different reasons for speech loss or impairment of the voice.

Stroke The loss of speech that can occur after a stroke will be sudden. Your relative may know what he wants, but be unable to communicate his needs, which can be very distressing. Often, he will literally have to be taught to speak again.

Voice box removal Someone who has had his voice box (*larynx*) removed will be more prepared for loss of speech. He may have a special device fitted that enables him to speak by modifying the sound produced by belching air from his stomach. This relearning process takes time and requires patience.

Brain damage Someone who is brain-damaged may be able to speak, but be unable to find the right word. This can be frustrating for both of you, but with patience you can learn to understand his needs.

GETTING SPECIALIST HELP

You may, in time, learn to recognise what your relative is trying to say, but it will help both of you if you seek the help of a specialist.

Ask to see a speech therapist A GP can refer your relative to a speech therapist, who is trained to recognise the nature of speech problems and how to overcome them. With his guidance, you will be able to help your relative with exercises, such as how to shape the mouth to form different sounds.

INDEPENDENCE AIDS

A person with impaired speech will be helped by having one or more of the items below to hand.

Pencil and paper
These should always be close to hand, so that your relative can write down requests.

Typing aids Specialist machines are available, or your relative could use a computer or typewriter to communicate his needs.

Visual aids He could hold up or point to images of frequently used items.

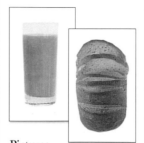

Pictures
Stick images from magazines on to cards.

INDEPENDENCE AIDS

Being registered blind (by an ophthalmologist) can provide entitlement to a range of special services and equipment. Contact the RNIB (*see page 175*) for information. Your relative should find out from his GP what is available on prescription.

Telling the time Clocks and watches with raised dots allow the person to tell the time.

Playing games Modified sets of popular games are available.

Reading and writing Braille is a system of printing in raised dots that can be read by touch. "Talking" books and large-print text also provide access to books.

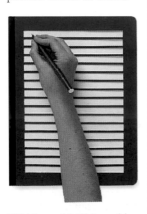

Writing aid This enables a visually impaired person to write in straight lines.

IMPAIRED SIGHT

This may be a condition present since birth, or it may come about as the result of disease or injury. If your relative's loss of sight is sudden, due, say, to an accident, it may be very frightening for him. If it develops gradually, you will both have time to get used to it and make the necessary adjustments. Where possible, try to help your relative to maintain independence. (*See also page 76*).

TYPES OF SIGHT LOSS

The level of impairment varies from person to person; few people have a complete lack of vision. Understanding the type of sight loss can enable you to help your relative. For instance, he may:

- ◆ distinguish only light;
- ◆ have no central vision;
- ◆ have no side vision;
- ◆ see only a vague blur;
- ◆ see only a mixture of blank spaces and defined areas.

COMMUNICATING WITH EACH OTHER

It is essential that your relative is independent and feels at ease in his home. The way you communicate with him is very important and may require you to adapt the way you would normally speak or respond. **Non-verbal signs** Avoid responding non-verbally, by nodding or shaking your head. Also, remember that body language, such as a smile or an outstretched hand, may be impossible for your relative to see. **Greetings and farewells** When you approach a blind person, always say "Hello" and take his hand to shake it or pat his arm or shoulder to reassure him. If you do not know him well, identify yourself. Tell him when you are leaving, so that he is not left talking to himself. **Talking** Do not change the way you speak. Do not be afraid to say "Nice to see you" – most blind people use this phrase themselves. If you and the person are in company, address him by name or use a light touch on the arm to indicate that you are speaking to him. **Personal space** To allow your relative maximum independence in the home, make sure his belongings and the items he frequently uses are kept in the same place; this will make it easier for him to locate things.

IMPAIRED HEARING

It is quite common for an elderly person's hearing to fail gradually. He may not realise that he is becoming deaf, or he may even refuse to accept his condition. Deafness may lead to feelings of isolation and rejection, and the person may think that people are talking about him or laughing at him behind his back. Try to be patient and reassuring.

COMMUNICATING WITH EACH OTHER

By reassessing the way in which you speak and the implications of your body language, you should be able to overcome the difficulties involved in communicating effectively.

Facing someone When you are talking to someone with impaired hearing, always face him so that he can lip-read what you are saying.

Tone of voice Learn to use the lower tones of your voice range, as someone with impaired hearing is more able to hear these.

Body language Use non-verbal communication as much as possible. Your body language (*see page 38*) may be an essential way of communicating with someone with impaired hearing.

Sign language If your relative is deaf, it is useful to learn sign language. You could also develop your own signs between you.

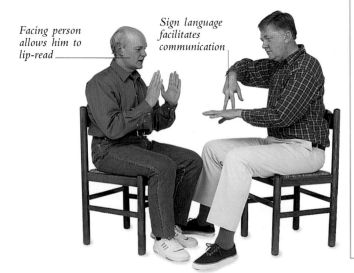

Facing person allows him to lip-read

Sign language facilitates communication

INDEPENDENCE AIDS

There is a range of aids available to help those with impaired hearing; information about these can be obtained from the RNID (*see page 175*). Before purchasing any aids, your relative should talk to his GP about what is available on prescription.

Hearing aid In order to ensure the hearing aid fits properly, a mould of your relative's ear will be taken. He should be warned that a hearing aid will magnify all sounds equally, so that he is prepared for this when he is in particularly noisy places. In order to work effectively, the hearing aid should not be allowed to get wet, and the batteries should be checked regularly.

Specialist telephones A variety of telephones are available; a flashing light can indicate ringing and some display the message on a screen.

Amplifying sound Personal amplifiers increase the sound of a radio or television. Portable amplifiers that attach to the earpiece of a telephone are also available.

DEALING WITH CONFUSION

I F A PERSON IS CONFUSED, he may forget simple facts, such as what day of the week it is, who someone is or his whereabouts. This can be frustrating for both of you and potentially dangerous for your relative. Although looking after a confused person requires patience, there are practical steps you can take to help him to remember things and become less dependent on you.

SHORT-TERM CONFUSION

Confusion is not always a long-term problem. Quite often, it can be a temporary condition – most commonly when the person is ill.

Due to illness
Sometimes an acute infection, for instance, can cause temporary confusion. You should give your relative plenty of fluids to prevent him from becoming dehydrated and help lessen the confusion. Consult the GP or district nurse for advice.

Drug-related
Confusion and behavioural changes may coincide with your relative being put on new medication. If this occurs, inform his GP of the problem so that a change of medication or dosage can be considered. Drug-related confusion can also occur when a person has been on long-term medication.

MEMORY LOSS

Confusion can cause or be the result of memory loss. Someone who has lost the ability to add to his long-term memory may forget something you said ten seconds ago, but be able to remember clearly an event that happened ten years ago. He may ask you the same question over and over again; not only has he forgotten the answer, he has probably forgotten that he ever asked you the question.

COMMUNICATING INFORMATION
You can help your relative by thinking about the way you communicate information.
Use active phrases Say, "It is time to take your tablets". Do not tell him hours before, "You need to take your tablets at three o'clock".
Be specific Be precise when writing a reminder: "Your hospital appointment is at 11am on Thursday, 16th May", not "Hospital appointment, Thursday".
Keep questions direct Ask your relative, "Would you like tea or coffee?" Do not ask him, "What would you like to drink?"

INDEPENDENCE AIDS
Use some of the methods recommended below to encourage independence. Discuss these with your relative first, as he may resent the house being cluttered with reminders telling him what to do.
Clocks and calendars All clocks and calendars should be correct; an alarm clock could be set to ring at the time your relative requires his medication.
Notice board List the things that are happening that day, such as visitors expected or outings planned.
Notes Place reminder notes, such as "Have you turned the oven off?" strategically.

CHAPTER 4

ADAPTING THE HOME

One of the main aims of caring is to help your
relative to maintain independence. To achieve this, it may be
necessary to make some changes to the home environment. This
chapter includes ideas for adapting every room in the home and
outlines the range of benefits that may be available to enable you
to do this. For example, if your relative uses a wheelchair
and an adaptation is essential to her quality of life, it is
possible that she would be awarded a grant.

WHAT YOU CAN DO

Adaptations should always be safe and, wherever possible,
also suitable for able-bodied members of the household.
Simple measures, such as rearranging furniture and moving
unnecessary clutter out of the way, can create space and allow
someone to move around more easily; giving thought to where
frequently needed items are placed can enable your relative to do
more for herself. If she has mobility problems or is wheelchair
bound, it may be necessary to obtain specialist equipment or make
structural changes, such as widening doors. It is essential that
you discuss any changes with your relative beforehand
and that she is happy with them, otherwise it could be
confusing for her to find things rearranged, especially if she has
been in hospital for some time.

GETTING HELP

ALWAYS SEEK THE ADVICE of an occupational therapist before embarking on any adaptations or purchasing specialist equipment. An occupational therapist is trained to assess the needs of the person you are caring for and advise on possible funding. A grant may be available if it is essential to purchase specialist equipment and/or make structural changes.

CASE STUDY

NAME: DOROTHY
AGE: 56

Dorothy, who is wheelchair bound due to a spinal injury, wanted to continue living in her flat. To enable her to do this, Social Services funded major adaptations to her kitchen and bathroom. However, some relatively minor problems still bothered her: for example, she couldn't get clothes out of the cupboard or reach plug sockets. She contacted a voluntary organisation who arranged for additional changes to be made, including moving door handles to the hinge side of the door (so that she did not have to lean too far out of her wheelchair to open it), lowering wardrobe rails and raising plug sockets. These small changes enabled Dorothy to be more independent and helped to improve her quality of life.

MAKING THE RIGHT ADAPTATIONS

Getting the right advice before you begin adapting the home is essential to your relative's safety and your own, and it can save you wasting time and money making changes that are of limited use.

SEEKING SPECIALIST HELP

Under the NHS and Community Care Act 1990, your relative is entitled to a free assessment of her situation; contact your local authority to arrange one. This may give you access to someone – usually an occupational therapist – who will:

◆ assess the needs of your relative;
◆ advise you on the best ways to adapt your home to suit your relative's needs;
◆ suggest specialist equipment that will enable your relative to live more independently;
◆ provide information on what financial support may be available.

If there is a delay, speak to the district nurse or GP who may be able to speed up the process. There are also independent disability services (*see page 177*) who can help and advise you on how to adapt your home, or put you in touch with an occupational therapist.

MAKING SHORT-TERM CHANGES

Your relative may be convalescing after an illness and her mobility, for example, may only be affected for a short amount of time. In this situation, look for practical and inexpensive ways to adapt your home. For example, instead of putting up an extra banister, would it be possible for your relative to sleep downstairs for a few weeks? If your relative needs specialist equipment for a short time, could you borrow it from a voluntary organisation?

Getting Financial help

Your local authority will be able to tell you whether you and your relative are eligible for financial benefits to meet the cost of purchasing specialist equipment or making essential structural changes. Even if you are not awarded a grant, your local authority is obliged to assist with changes that are "necessary for the greater convenience of the person"; some authorities will put up handrails or install ramps at no charge. You may be entitled to a grant, but remember:

- grants have to be approved before work can begin;
- the grant may not cover the full cost of the work.

Disabled facilities grant

The payment of this grant is compulsory if your relative is a disabled person who requires the use of specialist equipment, or structural changes to be made to the house, to be able to live more independently.
What does it cover? This grant covers changes required to improve access to any room, adaptations to the bathroom or toilet and alterations to lighting and heating controls. Grants for less essential requirements are awarded at the council's discretion.
How is a decision reached? The condition and structure of your home and your relative's ability to function are assessed. The assessor then recommends changes according to your relative's needs.
What amount of funding will be provided? This will depend on your relative's income and ability to pay.
How do I/we apply? You or your relative should contact the house renovation grants section of your local council. They are obliged to complete their assessment and give you a decision within six months of receipt of your application.

Minor works grants

These are available if your relative is over 60 and is claiming benefits. They are not available to council tenants and are awarded at the discretion of the council.
"Staying Put" grant This funds simple repairs or improvements to security and safety.
"Elderly Resident" grant This funds adaptations to your home that enable an elderly person to live with you permanently: installing an extra toilet, for example.

Buying Equipment

Most equipment can be obtained through mail-order companies, or a pharmacist may be able to order it. Disabled Living Centres and St John Ambulance and Red Cross depots also loan and sell equipment (*see pages 174–77*). Seek advice on the installation and use of all equipment.

Testing equipment
When purchasing expensive equipment, visit a Disabled Living Centre or Keep Able (*see page 177*) where you can examine and test the items on display. Manufacturers may come to your home to demonstrate very specialist equipment.

Second-hand equipment The Disabled Living Foundation (*see page 177*) has a fact sheet on where to find second-hand equipment; exercise more caution than when buying brand-new goods.

VAT Most equipment for disabled people and building costs for installing it are exempt from VAT. Fill in a form (usually available from the supplier) declaring the disability of the person.

GENERAL IMPROVEMENTS

I F A PERSON IS ILL OR HAS LIMITED MOBILITY, her quality of life may be greatly improved if she can get around the home easily and do things by herself. For example, simply rearranging furniture may be all she needs to be able to walk around safely and without your assistance. Look around your home for possible hazards, exercising great caution.

ADAPTATIONS AROUND THE HOME

For general safety, don't leave items lying around on the floor and tape down anything that is likely to cause your relative to trip, such as electrical flexes.
Flooring Remove rugs or secure them to the floor with double-sided tape. If your relative can't see very well, choose plain rather than patterned flooring.
Windows and curtains For those who are unable to stretch, long-handled catch openers to open windows, and curtains that have pulleys, are advised. You can

also get mains-operated devices.
Plugs and sockets Plugs with handles are useful for those with limited dexterity. Position sockets further up the wall for a wheelchair user.
Communication aids Intercom systems enable an immobile person to find out who is at the door and to communicate from another room. A panic button, attached to a help point, can also be installed. These are available from Age Concern (*see page 176*).

IMPROVING ACCESS INTO AND OUT OF THE HOME

Try to assess how easy it is for your relative to enter and leave the home, and make improvements, if possible.

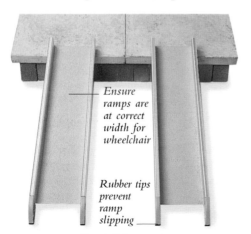

Ensure ramps are at correct width for wheelchair

Rubber tips prevent ramp slipping

Portable ramps

Gates or doors It may be necessary to widen gates or doors for wheelchair access – 80cm (32in) width is the minimum advised, but 100cm (40in) is preferable. Remove door sills, if possible, as these can be hazardous and impede people who are confined to wheelchairs, or those who use walking aids.
Garden access Pathways should be level or have only gentle slopes and be non-slip. They may need to be widened if wheelchair access is necessary. Also, don't put gravel down as this can make it difficult to move a wheelchair.
Ramps These can be installed over single steps for improved wheelchair access. You can get permanent ones or lightweight portable ones to make it easier to get into and out of the house.

HALLWAY AND STAIRS

To ENABLE YOUR RELATIVE TO get around the house with minimum effort, look particularly at the hallway and stairs. Hallways should be adapted to suit your relative's disability. Extra rails, or even a stairlift, can make all the difference to a disabled person who can't otherwise get up and down the stairs, and enable her to lead as normal a life as possible.

ADAPTING THE HALLWAY

Make sure that nothing in the hallway is preventing your relative from moving around with ease.

Lighting levels The hallway, landing and stairs should be well lit, especially for someone with impaired sight.

Furniture If your relative uses a wheelchair or walking frame around the house, keep the hallway as clear of furniture as possible. For someone who is unsteady on her feet, sturdy furniture in the hall may be useful as a support.

Grab rails Place these at appropriate places along the wall to help an immobile person to move along the hall.

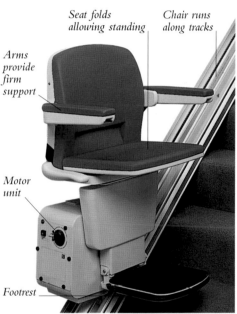

Seat folds *allowing standing*

Chair runs *along tracks*

Arms provide firm support

Motor unit

Footrest

Grab rail

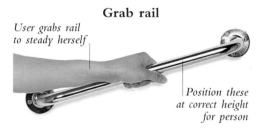

User grabs rail to steady herself

Position these at correct height for person

ADAPTING THE STAIRS

This may involve installing an extra banister or, more expensively, a lift.

Staircate A gate at the top and bottom of the stairs may help if the person suffers from confusion.

Banisters An extra banister placed along the wall makes it much easier for a person to get up or down stairs.

Stairlift A person who has difficulty climbing the stairs, or who is wheelchair bound, will benefit from the use of a stairlift. This is a "seat" attached to the staircase. The person sits in it and presses a button; it then moves slowly up or down the staircase.

Vertical through-floor lift This lift is installed in a ground-floor room and transports the person through a "trapdoor" in the ceiling to an upstairs room. It is very useful for wheelchair users who need a wheelchair upstairs, or where a stairlift cannot be fitted.

KITCHEN

To BE ABLE TO COOK BY HERSELF, your relative should have all the necessary kitchen facilities. This will reduce the burden on you, the carer, if you are the only person preparing meals. As well as making structural changes, you may need to obtain eating and drinking aids to help her to cook and prepare food as well as eat and drink by herself (*see page 68*).

ADAPTING THE KITCHEN

Consider simple changes, such as having an eating area in the kitchen so that your relative does not have to carry hot food to another room. Check that seating is comfortable and safe; a chair with arms is more suitable than a stool. If structural changes are necessary, opt for adaptations that will also suit members of the household who are able-bodied.

Lighting Strip lighting placed under wall units and shelves is especially useful for someone with impaired sight.

Cupboard and drawers Choose units with drawers that can be pulled right out so that all items can be accessed easily. Specialist cupboards with shelving that pulls out further are also available. If ordinary drawers and cupboards are being used, make sure frequently used items are easy to find.

Work surfaces If possible, fit pull-out work surfaces that are the correct height for a wheelchair user.

Cookers and ovens A hob guard offers protection from hot elements for the visually impaired. Control knobs positioned at the front of the cooker allow it to be operated without the person having to stretch over the hot hob.

Adjustable sink height

Trolley to transport hot items

High oven is ideal for someone who can't bend

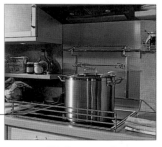

Guard prevents pan being knocked over

Hob guard

LIVING ROOM

THIS MAY BE THE ROOM where an inactive person spends most of her time. It should be made as comfortable as possible, so that she can enjoy her leisure time independently. It is important to get the right type of chair for her to sit in: one that she is comfortable in and that she can get into and out of fairly easily. Make sure that she has everything she needs to hand.

ADAPTING THE LIVING ROOM

If your relative has mobility problems, she should be seated in the best position in the room. Ideally, sit her by the window so that she can see outside, but ensure that she is shaded from direct sunlight.

Footrest This can provide comfort for someone who is seated. A bean bag is an ideal footrest.

Remote control systems Get your relative a television or stereo that has a remote control so that she is able to operate it from her chair. Those who have very limited mobility can even get remote-controlled curtains and lights.

BUYING A CHAIR

If you are purchasing a chair for someone who is weak or immobile, choose one that has firm arms and a high seat so it is easier for her to get into and out of by herself. Alternatively, there is a variety of specialist chairs that can be self-operated to raise the user to a standing position.

Mechanical chair

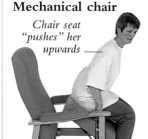

Chair seat "pushes" her upwards

User presses lever

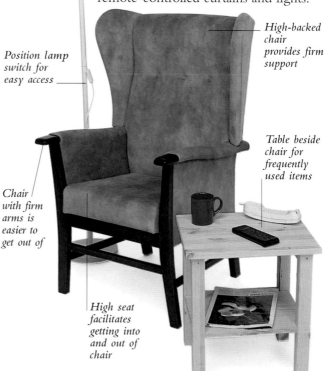

Position lamp switch for easy access

Chair with firm arms is easier to get out of

High-backed chair provides firm support

Table beside chair for frequently used items

High seat facilitates getting into and out of chair

BATHROOM AND TOILET

I F YOUR RELATIVE NEEDS YOUR HELP to wash and use the toilet, it may be embarrassing for her and time-consuming for you. It may help to get the bathroom and toilet altered so that she can use them by herself. It is also worth considering how difficult it is for her to reach the bathroom and toilet, and, if possible, make the route easier. (*See also* Personal Care, *pages 97–106*).

ADAPTING THE BATHROOM AND TOILET

Some alterations to the layout of the bathroom and toilet are essential for safety. An ideal layout is shown below, but you may find that a rail or a frame around the toilet is all that is necessary.

Bathroom or toilet door Sliding or folding doors allow easier wheelchair access and may also enable you to reach a person who has fallen more easily.

Flooring Fitted carpet is safer than a tiled or lino floor, which can be slippery when the floor is wet.

Frames or grab rails Fitted around the toilet, bath or shower, these can provide enough support to allow a weak person to use them alone.

TOILET SEAT

The toilet seat can be raised to help a weak person to get on and off it more easily. This can be done by installing a base under the toilet or by fitting a raised toilet seat. These seats fit on most standard toilets and are removable so that they can be washed.

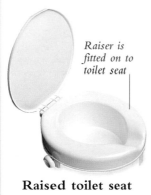

Raiser is fitted on to toilet seat

Raised toilet seat

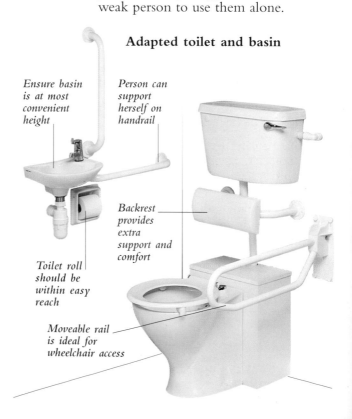

Adapted toilet and basin

Ensure basin is at most convenient height

Person can support herself on handrail

Backrest provides extra support and comfort

Toilet roll should be within easy reach

Moveable rail is ideal for wheelchair access

SINKS

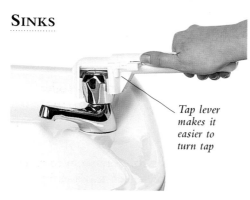

Tap lever makes it easier to turn tap

Taps Those with cross tops are easier to operate than rounded ones, which can be difficult to grip. You can install replacement lever taps, or fit temporary levers. These enable a person with weak hands or wrists to turn the tap on and off with ease.

Sink height Sinks may need to be lowered for a wheelchair user or raised if a person cannot bend easily.

BATHS AND SHOWERS

To enable your relative to wash herself, you may have to adapt your bath or shower. To prevent accidents, place a mat inside (*see below*) and beside the bath. Avoid using bath oils as these can cause a hazardous surface.

Bath seat This can be placed in the bath when your relative wants to use it (*see page 98*). Mechanical seats called "bath-lifters", that can be self-operated, are also available.

Shower cubicle If a person has difficulty getting into a bath, a shower cubicle is often a simpler option. Shower units with level or ramped access, instead of sills that have to be stepped or wheeled over, are much easier to use. Ensure that the shower has non-slip flooring, or use a mat.

Shower seat This can be placed in the shower cubicle and is useful for someone who is too weak to stand. A chair that can be wheeled into the shower is also available, but door sills may have to be removed if this is used.

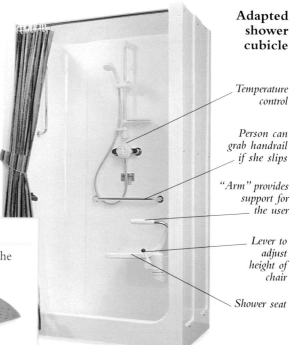

Adapted shower cubicle

Temperature control

Person can grab handrail if she slips

"Arm" provides support for the user

Lever to adjust height of chair

Shower seat

NON-SLIP MATS

A non-slip mat should be placed in the bath or shower to prevent a person slipping when she gets in and out.

Pads on bottom grip surface

BEDROOM

I F THE MAJORITY OF PRACTICAL CARE is carried out in this room, there must be sufficient space around the bed to carry out procedures safely and easily. It may also be necessary to raise a low bed. If your relative can get out of bed but has mobility problems, you may need to adapt her wardrobe so that she can get her clothes more easily. (*See also* Bed Comfort, *pages 83–96*).

ADAPTING THE BEDROOM

This room should be comfortable and easy to use, especially for someone who is confined to bed for long periods. Light switches and lamps should be near the bed – select an angled lamp if the person likes to read in bed. If a toilet aid is used (*see page 114*), keep this near the bed. Place a suitable chair next to the bed for your relative to sit in and for visitors.

Cupboard doors and shelving Wardrobes with sliding doors and pull-out shelving enable someone who has difficulty stretching to access clothes.

Wardrobes Lowering rails and handles helps a wheelchair user to reach clothes.
Television and radio Obtain equipment that has a remote control.

BED RAISERS

These can be attached to the legs of a low bed to raise it so that it is easier for the person to get into and out of, and to minimise any risk of back strain to you. Seek the advice of a healthcare professional about which type to use and fit them securely.

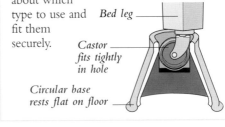

Bed leg

Castor fits tightly in hole

Circular base rests flat on floor

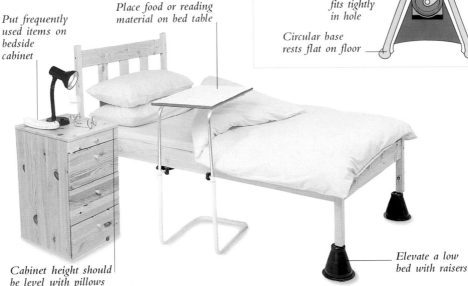

Put frequently used items on bedside cabinet

Place food or reading material on bed table

Cabinet height should be level with pillows

Elevate a low bed with raisers

CHAPTER 5

HOME HYGIENE

If your relative is ill or frail, or is taking
certain medication, he may be particularly vulnerable
to infection, so it is essential to maintain as hygienic and
germ-free an environment as possible. It is also important to
protect yourself from infection, because if you become ill, not
only will you be unable to fulfil your role efficiently, you may
also put the health of your relative at risk.

CLEANLINESS

There are many preventive measures you can
take to eliminate germs (*bacteria* and *viruses*) and minimise the
spread of infection. The most important of these measures is to
maintain a high standard of personal hygiene: a simple task such as
handwashing is often done in a quick, perfunctory
way, but washing your hands thoroughly is an essential
part of basic cleanliness.

DISPOSAL OF WASTE

If your relative is ill or incontinent, part of your
caring role may include dealing with the disposal of his body
waste, such as blood, faeces, vomit or urine.
It is essential that you follow the correct procedures for the
disposal of this waste to minimise the risk of infecting
yourself, and to prevent any infection from
spreading to other people.

INFECTION AND ITS CAUSES

AN INFECTION IS THE RESULT of the body being invaded by germs (*bacteria* and *viruses*). This causes an adverse reaction – directly by damaging cells, or indirectly by releasing poisonous substances (*toxins*) into the body. The symptoms will depend on the type of infection, where it is located and whether it has spread throughout the body.

THE SYMPTOMS OF INFECTION

The symptoms of an infection depend on whether the infection is confined to one area or has spread throughout the body (*see opposite* and *pages 178–80*). For example, an infection caused by an abscess may be localised, whereas the infection caused by chickenpox, measles or a common cold will affect the whole body.

Symptoms of a localised infection may be:
◆ pain and swelling;
◆ localised redness;
◆ loss of movement;
◆ areas that are hot to the touch.

Symptoms of an infection throughout the body may be:
◆ high temperature and increased breathing and pulse rates (*see page 128*);
◆ headache and thirst;
◆ hot, dry skin and rash;
◆ loss of appetite;
◆ weakness and apathy.

HOW INFECTION SPREADS

An infection is only dangerous if it is given a suitable environment in which to flourish.

Sources People and animals are the sources of most infections, carrying many bacteria and viruses.

Routes An infection can be passed on through direct and indirect routes (*see below*).

Victim Anyone can become infected, but the most vulnerable are those who have not been vaccinated, and those who have low immunity (*see page 56*), such as a frail person or someone in poor health.

DIRECT AND INDIRECT ROUTES

A person can catch an infection *directly* by touching something that is contaminated; by sharing a needle with a contaminated person; through an exchange of body fluids such as blood or saliva; or through sexual activity with an infected person. An infection can be spread *indirectly* in a variety of ways.

Airborne Germs can be carried in the droplets of fluid expelled when coughing and sneezing.

Food This can become contaminated if it is not stored, handled or cooked correctly (*see page 60*).

Clothing or equipment These can harbour germs if they are not cleaned regularly and thoroughly.

Insects A number of insects, especially house flies, can spread infection.

TREATING INFECTION

If you suspect that you or your relative has an infection, seek medical help as soon as possible. The GP may prescribe a course of antibiotics for bacterial infections; these will only be effective if the course is completed. If the infection is viral, the GP will usually only be able to treat the symptoms.

SOME INFECTIOUS DISEASES (see also pages 178–80)

DISEASE	POSSIBLE SIGNS AND SYMPTOMS	HOW IT MAY BE TRANSMITTED	INFECTIOUS PERIOD
Gastro-enteritis	Appetite loss, nausea, vomiting, diarrhoea, abdominal cramps.	Contaminated food or water supplies.	Up to two days after diarrhoea stops.
Glandular fever	Fever, headache, swollen glands in neck, armpits and groin, severe sore throat, fatigue.	Contact with saliva.	Variable – may be weeks.
Hepatitis A, B, C, D and E	Flu-like illness, followed by jaundice. Some people have no symptoms.	A, E: infected food or water; B, C, D: sexually transmitted; contaminated blood; shared needles.	A, E: one week after jaundice. B, C, D: varies; blood can be infectious for life.
Herpes simplex (cold sores and genital herpes)	Small, fluid-filled, irritating blisters, slight temperature.	Contact with lesions.	Until blisters crust over.
Herpes zoster (chickenpox and shingles)	Chickenpox: slight fever, groups of itchy, dark red spots that become blisters. Shingles: localised, painful blistering rash.	Airborne; contact with rash.	Until all blisters crust over.
HIV/AIDS	May be symptomless for years; breathlessness, fever, weight loss, diarrhoea, swollen glands and fatigue may eventually occur.	Sexually transmitted; contaminated blood; shared needles; mother to child.	For life.
Influenza, common cold	Fever, cough, runny nose, headache, sore throat, chills, aches, pains.	Airborne.	First few days.
Meningitis	Fever, headache, drowsiness, confusion, rash, reaction to light.	Various methods, usually airborne.	A week before and ten days after fever.
Tuber-culosis	Fever, cough, swollen and painful glands, stiff neck, weight loss.	Airborne.	While phlegm is infected.

PREVENTING INFECTION

THE BODY'S IMMUNE SYSTEM cannot fully protect against infection. It is essential, therefore, for your own health and that of your relative, to take steps to eliminate the germs that cause infection from your home environment. The risks can be minimised if you maintain a good level of cleanliness and take proper precautions when dealing with body waste.

PERSONAL HYGIENE

You can maintain a high standard of cleanliness, and minimise the risk of infection, by washing your hands thoroughly and wearing disposable gloves. It is important that you follow the correct technique for removing gloves once they are soiled.

THE BODY'S NATURAL DEFENCES

The immune system is the body's main defence against infection. White blood cells circulate around the body and destroy harmful bacteria. People with leukaemia, for example, who have a low number of these cells, will be more prone to infection.

WASHING YOUR HANDS THOROUGHLY

Wash your hands before and after preparing food, after using the toilet and before and after giving care, even if gloves are worn. Scrub dirty nails as part of your handwashing routine.

1 Wet and soap your hands. Rub your palms together to form a lather.

To clean thoroughly, build up rich lather

2 Rub the palm and fingers of one hand over the back of the other, interlocking the fingers. Repeat for the other hand.

Clean back of hand and between fingers

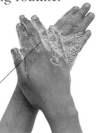

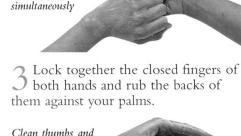

Clean palms and backs of fingers simultaneously

3 Lock together the closed fingers of both hands and rub the backs of them against your palms.

Clean thumbs and fronts of fingers simultaneously

4 Clean each thumb by rubbing it against the fronts of your fingers.

5 Clean your fingertips by rubbing them on the palm of the opposite hand. This also cleans the palm.

6 Rinse your hands and dry them on a clean cloth or paper towel.

Wearing and removing gloves

Gloves should be worn whenever a procedure involves contact with body fluids, and when creams or lotions are being applied. To prevent any substance coming into contact with your skin, always remove gloves following the procedure below. Disposable latex or vinyl gloves are available from most chemists. The thinner, polythene varieties should not be used as they do not provide adequate protection.

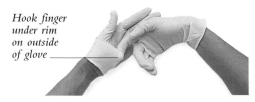

Hook finger under rim on outside of glove

1 Pick up the base of the left-hand glove with your right index finger. Pull it halfway off your hand, leaving the top half of your thumb covered.

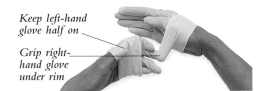

Keep left-hand glove half on

Grip right-hand glove under rim

2 Repeat step 1 to remove the glove on your right hand, but this time pull the glove all the way off, so that it is completely inside out.

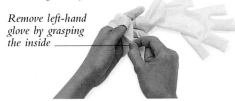

Remove left-hand glove by grasping the inside

3 Use your now uncovered right hand to pull the left glove off, so that both gloves are now inside out.

4 Pick up the gloves on the inside and dispose of them safely.

Cleaning Equipment

Some of the items used when caring may be disposable, but others will require thorough cleaning.

Toilet aids (*see page 114*) Clean bedpans, urinals and commode pans with hot, soapy water.

Thermometers (*see pages 126–28*) Before use, rinse the thermometer in cold water and dry it with a paper towel. After use, wipe it with a damp cloth or cotton wool.

Washing accessories Wash flannels and towels regularly. It is advisable to use separate towels and flannels on the face and body.

Surfaces Clean surfaces such as table-tops and bed-trays with a detergent, and dry thoroughly with a clean cloth.

Containing your own Germs

It is particularly important to take steps to ensure that you do not spread your own germs to your relative.

Illness If you are ill, it will not be beneficial to you or your relative if you continue caring. Inform a care professional so that alternative arrangements can be made (*see pages 24–25*).

Coughing and sneezing Use a tissue or handkerchief and avoid coughing or sneezing in the direction of your relative.

Skin infections If you have cuts, abrasions or a skin disorder, you must ensure that the entire area is properly protected by gloves or a waterproof dressing before giving care.

NEEDLE AND SYRINGE DISPOSAL

If a medication has to be given by injection, or your relative has to test his blood through pin-pricks, the safe disposal of needles and syringes is essential. These should be placed in a British Standards Approved container, called a "sharps" box, which is supplied by local health services, but is also available from chemists. A healthcare professional will arrange to collect and dispose of the box at regular agreed intervals. Follow these guidelines:

◆ keep the sharps box out of the reach of children as they may be able to access the needles;

◆ do not fill the box beyond the three-quarters level;

◆ do not place the box in a domestic bin-bag.

Sharps box

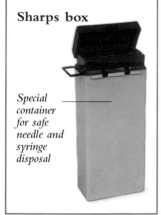

Special container for safe needle and syringe disposal

DISPOSING OF BODY WASTE

When you are caring for someone, you should take precautions to prevent yourself, and anyone else, from coming into contact with that person's body waste. The risk of spreading infection can be greatly reduced if you take the necessary preventive measures. When disposing of waste, wear latex gloves and an apron, if available. If you are caring for someone who is known to be suffering from a blood-borne infection, such as HIV or hepatitis, seek advice from the person's GP.

METHODS OF DISPOSAL

There are two safe ways to dispose of waste.
Down the toilet Place body fluids and soiled tissues in the toilet bowl, close the lid and flush the toilet twice.
In a plastic bag Some waste materials, such as dressings and incontinence pads, should be placed in a secure plastic bag, which must be sealed before being placed in the rubbish bin – never flush them down the toilet. If your relative has a blood-borne infection, official yellow plastic bags will be supplied and collected for incineration.

CLEANING SPILLAGES

Wear latex gloves, cover the body waste with paper towels and pour undiluted bleach over the towels if the waste is on a hard surface. Gather it all up with clean paper towels and dispose of it in a sealed plastic bag. If the spill is on a carpet, use hot, soapy water, not bleach.

NEEDLESTICK INJURY

If you accidentally prick yourself with a used needle, or other sharp object that has come into contact with body fluids, do not suck the injury to stop it from bleeding. To prevent the spread of infection, follow this procedure:

◆ wash the affected area under cold, running water;

◆ encourage the wound to bleed freely;

◆ inform your GP or other healthcare professional.

If you are a volunteer carer, you must inform the organisation for whom you are working so that the incident can be documented.

CHAPTER 6

HEALTHY EATING & DRINKING

Your relative may have a small appetite or find eating difficult
because of an illness, a disability or general apathy, but it is
essential that she is encouraged to eat well and regularly. Achieving
a balanced diet is always possible, even if someone has to follow a
special diet for health or personal reasons. To help you to meet the
requirements of a balanced diet, this chapter provides a basic
understanding of nutrition.

MAKING MEALTIMES ENJOYABLE

To make mealtimes enjoyable and relaxed, try to gain
an understanding of your relative's needs and, if she is physically
impaired, find practical ways that allow her to be more
independent when eating or drinking. Simple measures can
be taken to make meals look and taste as appetising as possible;
this is especially important for someone who is
ill and does not have a strong appetite.

CARING FOR YOURSELF

As a carer it is easy to neglect your own needs and get
into bad habits, such as skipping meals or snacking. To meet the
high energy demands required for caring, however, it is essential
that you also eat sensibly and regularly (*see page 19*).

HYGIENE IN THE KITCHEN

SOMEONE WHO IS ILL OR FRAIL may be particularly vulnerable to infection. It is, therefore, essential to take simple steps when preparing and cooking food to reduce the risk of contamination. In order to minimise any health risks, you need to keep your kitchen and cooking utensils clean, shop sensibly, store food wisely and prepare it carefully.

DO'S & DON'TS

Follow these guidelines when you are buying and storing food:

☑ **Do** check that the inner wrapping of packaged goods, and the seals and rims of tinned goods, are not damaged.

☑ **Do** check the expiry date on goods before purchasing them.

☑ **Do** put food in the fridge or freezer as soon as possible after purchase.

☑ **Do** place fruit and vegetables in the bottom of the fridge, and fish and meat in the coldest part. Clean out fridges and freezers regularly.

☒ **Don't** store raw and cooked foods on the same shelf. Put raw meat and defrosting products on a plate to stop them from dripping.

☒ **Don't** put raw and frozen foods in the same shopping bag. Place frozen food in a cool bag, if you have one.

HYGIENE TIPS

To prevent food contamination, make the following simple steps part of your daily routine when using your kitchen and preparing and cooking meals.

CLEANLINESS
- Keep pets away from all food and kitchen surfaces.
- Wash your hands before and after preparing food.
- Clean utensils and cutting tools thoroughly.
- Change and wash cloths and towels regularly.
- Avoid wiping your hands repeatedly on an apron or cloth; do not use tea towels as hand towels.
- Cover any cuts or sores on your hands.

PREPARATION
- Do not eat food from damaged containers, or food that has passed its expiry date.
- Wash fresh fruit and vegetables thoroughly.
- Do not use the same knife or chopping board to prepare cooked and uncooked foods at the same time.
- Do not prepare food too far in advance.
- Follow frozen food guidelines carefully.

COOKING
- Ensure that all meat and fish is thoroughly cooked.
- Do not taste food with your fingers.
- When reheating food, check that it is thoroughly hot and do not reheat it more than once.
- Follow cooking guidelines exactly on all products.
- Eat cooked food while it is hot.
- Avoid giving the following foods to the ill or the elderly: pâté or soft cheeses, as these may contain listeria bacteria; raw eggs, under-cooked eggs or under-cooked meat, especially poultry, as these can cause salmonella poisoning.

EATING A BALANCED DIET

To MAINTAIN GOOD HEALTH you need to eat the right balance of foods from each of the five main food groups (*see page 63*), and drink plenty of fluids. Provided no particular food is eaten to excess, and sufficient calories are consumed for the body's daily needs (2750 calories for a physically active man, 2000 for a physically active woman), your diet should be well balanced.

WHAT YOUR BODY NEEDS

Your body needs a combination of nutrients – proteins, carbohydrates, fats, vitamins, minerals and fibre – to satisfy all its requirements.

PROTEINS

Proteins supply the body with the amino acids that are required to build new protein. Animal foods provide all the essential amino acids, while plant foods need to be combined (*see page 64*).

CARBOHYDRATES

These are starches or sugars and are the body's main source of energy. Starches are broken down into single molecules by the digestive system before being absorbed into the bloodstream, and often contain beneficial fibre (*see below*). Sugars are absorbed rapidly, supplying an instant, but short-term, surge of energy.

FATS

These are a good energy source (especially for those who have high energy requirements, such as the elderly) and are an essential component of the body's cells. However, saturated fat in particular should be eaten in moderation, due to the risk of heart disease and obesity.

VITAMINS AND MINERALS

These are an essential part of a balanced diet; they help the body to function properly and contribute to overall good health.

FIBRE

This passes through the body unchanged and is essential in preventing bowel and digestive problems. Fibre is also filling and may, therefore, reduce calorie intake.

FOOD SOURCES

Where to find the food types contained in a balanced diet.

Animal foods Meat, poultry, fish, eggs, milk and cheese.

Plant foods Bread, pasta, potatoes, rice, beans and pulses.

Starches Potatoes, bread, rice, pasta and some fruit.

Sugars Table sugar, sweets, biscuits and jam.

Unsaturated fats Oily fish, some vegetable oils and margarine.

Saturated fats Red meat, full-fat milk and other dairy products.

Vitamins and minerals These are found in a variety of foods (*see overleaf*). A balanced diet should prevent the need for supplements.

Fibre Wholemeal bread, cereals, potatoes, peas, bananas, oranges and green vegetables.

WHAT VITAMINS CAN DO

VITAMIN	WHAT IT DOES	WHERE IT CAN BE FOUND
A	Enhances normal growth, night vision, protects against infection.	Liver, fish-liver oils, egg yolk, dairy products, margarine, oranges, carrots.
Vitamin B complex, including B1, B2, B6	Promotes breakdown of fats, carbohydrates and proteins. Helps to form important body constituents, such as heart and body muscle.	Pasta, bran, wholemeal bread, meat, eggs, beans, cereals.
B12	Helps to form red blood cells and to keep the nervous system healthy.	Offal, chicken, fish, eggs, dairy products.
C	Maintains healthy bones and teeth; aids iron absorption.	Vegetables, fruit, especially citrus fruit, potatoes.
D	Essential for strong bones and teeth; helps calcium absorption.	Oily fish, liver, milk, egg yolk, margarine; in skin from sunlight.
E	Aids formation of red blood cells; slows down cell ageing.	Vegetable oils, nuts, meat, green vegetables, cereals.
K	Promotes blood clotting.	Green vegetables, vegetable oils, cheese, pork, liver.

WHAT MINERALS CAN DO

MINERAL	WHAT IT DOES	WHERE IT CAN BE FOUND
Sodium	A constituent of salt, it helps to hold water in the body.	Salt, bread, cereals, bacon, ham.
Potassium	Regulates the heart; helps the function of the nervous system and kidneys.	Meat, milk, fruit, vegetables.
Calcium	Helps blood to clot and keeps bones and teeth healthy.	Milk, green leafy vegetables, beans.
Iron	A constituent of the oxygen-carrying pigment of red blood cells.	Liver, meat, egg yolk, wholegrain cereal, nuts, beans.
Fluoride	Helps to harden the teeth and strengthen the bones.	Fish, tea, coffee, soya beans; sometimes added to water.
Iodine	Aids action of thyroid gland, which controls growth and development.	Salt-water fish, shellfish.

EATING FROM THE FIVE MAIN FOOD GROUPS

To maintain a balanced diet, you need to choose a combination of foods from the five main food groups. The chart below is a guide to the types of food in each group and the nutrients they provide. It also includes the recommended guidelines for what you should eat daily and gives tips on how to increase or decrease your intake of particular types of foods.

THE MAIN FOOD GROUPS

FOOD GROUP	WHAT IT CONTAINS	DAILY NEEDS
Cereals and potatoes	**Bread, pasta, oats, cereal, potatoes and rice** Good sources of starch and energy; rich in fibre, vitamins and minerals.	**Four portions** Boost your intake by eating all types, and opt for high-fibre varieties where possible. Try not to eat them with added fat.
Fruit and vegetables	**Fruit and vegetables** These are a good source of vitamins, minerals and fibre. Fresh is best, but frozen, dried and tinned can also be eaten.	**Four or five portions** Eat some fruit and vegetables raw. A glass of fruit juice is one serving. Check tinned products for added salt or sugar.
Meat, fish and alternatives	**Fish, nuts, meat, eggs, poultry, soya and seeds** These foods are good sources of protein, vitamins and minerals.	**Two portions** Choose lean cuts of meat, and fish such as salmon and herring. Remove the skin from poultry to reduce the fat content.
Milk and dairy products	**Cheese, yogurt and cream** Good sources of calcium and protein, but many products from this group have a high saturated fat content.	**Two portions** Choose low-fat varieties, such as semi-skimmed milk, low-fat yogurt and cheeses such as Edam.
Fatty and sugary foods	**Jam, butter, sweets, chocolate, oil, sugar and crisps** These are high in calories and provide the body with energy, but many contain saturated fats.	**Eat only occasionally** This is the only group that should not be eaten every day. Only eat these foods in small quantities. Try snacking on fruit and vegetables instead.

SPECIAL DIETS

Y OU MAY HAVE TO ADAPT your relative's diet for health reasons or to satisfy her personal tastes. Always follow the advice of a nutritionist or doctor if your relative's diet is restricted for medical reasons, and respect your relative's wishes if she chooses not to eat certain foods. Whatever types of food you are providing, try to meet the requirements of a balanced diet.

COMBINING PLANT FOODS

Unlike animal foods, no single plant food contains all the amino acids that the body requires. To assist their intake of "complete" proteins, therefore, non-meat eaters need to make sure that they eat plant foods in the correct combinations.

Good combinations

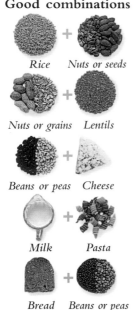

Rice + *Nuts or seeds*

Nuts or grains + *Lentils*

Beans or peas + *Cheese*

Milk + *Pasta*

Bread + *Beans or peas*

A DIET FOR HEALTH REASONS

Certain illnesses and conditions can result in dietary restrictions. For example, someone with heart disease may have to reduce salt or fat intake, and a condition such as diabetes may necessitate a controlled sugar intake. A GP or nutritionist will be able to advise on what can and cannot be eaten.

A VEGETARIAN DIET

Vegetarians do not eat meat or fish. Most will eat some animal foods, such as dairy produce, but always check the person's preference. A vegetarian diet differs from a non-vegetarian one in several ways.
A low level of saturated fat Because of the absence of red meat in a vegetarian diet, the level of saturated fat content will be low.
A high level of fibre The diet is more likely to contain meat alternatives, such as beans, pulses and grains, and will therefore be high in fibre.
Incomplete proteins There will be a lack of complete proteins due to the absence of meat in the diet (*see left*).

A VEGAN DIET

A person on a vegan diet does not eat meat or dairy products, but uses milk, butter and cheese made from nuts and soya beans. Like vegetarians, vegans need to combine a range of plant foods in order to ensure that they are getting sufficient proteins (*see left*). Due to the absence of certain foods from their diet, they may also need to take vitamin pill supplements (especially B12). If you are unsure whether or not vitamins are needed, consult a GP or nutritionist.

CULTURAL DIETS

As a volunteer carer, you may be looking after someone whose beliefs are different from your own, so it is essential to understand their dietary needs. Fasting may be required on certain days, but in most cultures the infirm, elderly and babies are excluded from this, especially if the fast involves fluid deprivation. The actual dates for fasting may change from year to year.

SPECIAL CULTURAL REQUIREMENTS		
CULTURE	DIETARY PREFERENCES	RESTRICTIONS
Hindu	◆ Many Hindus are vegetarian. ◆ Beef is never eaten. ◆ Cow's milk is acceptable. ◆ Fasting is common, although fruit, salad without salt, and hot milk or tea are allowed.	◆ May object to utensils that have been used to prepare meat or meat products. ◆ Alcohol and tobacco are forbidden. **Special days in calendar:** Fasting on *Ramanavami* (1 day), *Dushera* (10 days) and *Karva Chauth* (1 day).
Islam	◆ Halal meat (from animals that have been ritually slaughtered according to Muslim law) is eaten. ◆ Muslims do not eat pork or meat from other carnivorous animals.	◆ Halal meat should be stored and cooked separately from other products. ◆ Alcohol and tobacco are forbidden. **Special days in calendar:** Fasting during *Ramadan* (30 days) from dawn to dusk, and *Shab-E-Barat* (1 day) three weeks before *Ramadan* begins.
Jewish	◆ Kosher meat (blessed by a Rabbi and killed in a certain way) is preferred. ◆ Orthodox Jews avoid pork, bacon, ham, rabbit and shellfish. ◆ Meat and poultry must not be served with dairy products.	◆ Separate utensils must be used for dairy and meat products. ◆ Three hours should elapse between eating meat and any dairy product. **Special days in calendar:** Fasting on *Yom Kippur* (25 hours) and food restrictions for Passover (8 days).
Sikhs	◆ Dairy produce is important. ◆ Beef is never eaten. ◆ Many Sikhs are vegetarian, but some can eat meat slaughtered following a rite called *Chakardi*.	◆ Alcohol and tobacco are forbidden. **Special days in calendar:** Some people, often women, fast; they do not avoid all foods, but may reduce the quantity or variety of food eaten for one to two days per week.
Chinese	◆ Believe that health is related to a balance of the body's physical elements (*Taoism*).	◆ May think that cold food should not be eaten by an ill person or that an illness indicates a need to alter the diet.

MAKING MEALTIMES ENJOYABLE

IDEALLY, A BALANCED DIET is made up of three meals a day but, if this is not possible, you should try to provide the equivalent amount of food and correct combination of nutrients on a daily basis. To encourage your relative to eat meals, try to provide appetising food in a relaxed environment, and make sure she has the necessary items to enable her to eat without assistance.

PROVIDING FOOD FOR AN ILL PERSON

If your relative is ill, she may have little or no appetite. With short-term illnesses, such as a cold or mild flu, eating less is acceptable provided fluid intake is maintained. For long-term illnesses, however, the right amount of food and the correct balance of nutrients is essential to help the body to fight disease and repair damage. If you are worried about the level of your relative's food intake, her GP may suggest food supplements.

Quantity of food If your relative has lost her appetite, three large meals a day may prove daunting. It is better for her to eat a few small meals than to feel defeated because she cannot finish what is on her plate. Give her small, manageable portions throughout the day, and remove any leftovers immediately. Be patient and encouraging.

PREPARING FOR A MEAL

To maximise enjoyment, make sure that your relative is comfortable and that she has everything she needs to hand. She should have enough room in which to eat her meal – whether she is sitting in a chair, or using a tray or bed table – and the food should look and taste as appetising as possible.

PROVIDE A RELAXED ENVIRONMENT
Listen to your relative's wishes: she may want music, or the television or radio turned on during her meal. Check whether she would like to use the toilet before eating, and offer her a chance to freshen up. You may want to consider freshening the room with flowers or potpourri. Eating in company can be more enjoyable than eating alone so, if it is convenient, you, or other members of the household, should join your relative for a meal.

ENSURE MEALS ARE APPETISING
Where possible, your relative should help to decide what is going to be cooked and, if she is able, be encouraged to help prepare the meal.
Think about what you give her Provide foods that she enjoys – and that she is allowed to eat – in small, manageable portions.
Make the food attractive Presentation is important with any meal and can encourage someone, who may otherwise have little appetite, to eat. Provide a choice of seasoning and pickles, but remember that some items, such as salt, may not be permitted because of a medical condition (*see page 64*). If it does not conflict with dietary restrictions, an alcoholic drink, such as a glass of sherry or wine before or with a meal, may stimulate her appetite.

Adapting for a Physical Impairment

Physical impairment does not necessarily mean that your relative cannot feed herself or enjoy her meals. You can encourage independence by obtaining special aids to suit her specific needs (*see overleaf*).

Someone without teeth
If your relative is not able to wear dentures, she will find it difficult to chew, and will require a diet of soft foods. Prepare foods that can be mashed or use a mincer or liquidiser, if available.

Someone who is bedridden
Make a bedridden person as comfortable as possible, using pillows to aid sitting. Place the items on a bed table or tray (*see page 86*) and check that the bedclothes are properly protected.

Someone who cannot feed herself
If it is necessary to feed your relative, you can help to create a more relaxed atmosphere by talking and making her feel more comfortable. If you behave naturally, it will help to make both of you feel less self-conscious. When offering the food, make sure you hold the fork or spoon in your relative's line of vision so that she is able to see what she is eating.

Catering Help

If you are unable to provide meals, perhaps due to illness or because you are away from the house in the daytime, you may be able to get outside help. Seek advice from a care professional to find out what services are available in your area.

Meals on Wheels This service provides a regular midday meal from Monday to Friday (and sometimes at weekends). A financial contribution may be required for each meal.

Day centres If your relative attends a day centre, it is likely that she will be provided with a midday meal.

Helping a Visually Impaired Person

Someone who is visually impaired should be able to feed herself, but thoughtful preparation will be required to enable her to be independent. Think about what you prepare – foods such as peas, for example, may be difficult for the person to eat as they slide around the plate.

The "clock" method By simply arranging the food on the plate in a certain way, a visually impaired person can have more control over what she is choosing to eat. If she is told where the food is on the plate – for example, the potatoes are at "12 o' clock" – she will be able to eat without your assistance.

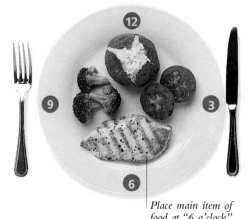

Place main item of food at "6 o'clock"

Aids to Eating and Drinking

SPECIALIST AIDS CAN ENABLE SOMEONE who has restricted use of an arm or a hand to prepare food for herself, and eat and drink without help. These aids range from devices that enable a person to open containers and prepare food, to specially adapted crockery and cutlery. The kitchen may also need to be adapted to suit the person's needs (*see page 48*).

Preparing Food

Cutting and spreading aids
Devices that hold food in place are available. For example, bread can be secured while it is spread with butter or sliced. These items are very useful for someone who can use only one hand.

Cooking basket
Lifting hot pans can be dangerous for someone who is frail or has a weak grip. By using a cooking basket, the person can lower the food into the hot water and, when it is cooked, simply lift the basket out of the water without having to lift the pan.

Opening Jars and Bottles

Jar openers
A variety of openers with grooves or bands to grip the lids of bottles and jars are available. The openers enable someone with weak hands or wrists to open jars more easily.

Using a grooved jar opener

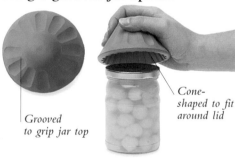

Grooved to grip jar top

Cone-shaped to fit around lid

Using an expandable jar opener

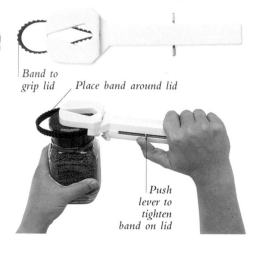

Band to grip lid   *Place band around lid*

Push lever to tighten band on lid

Pasta is lowered into boiling water

Using a cooking basket

DRINKING AIDS

Cups Drinking from a normal cup can be difficult and dangerous for someone who has a weak grip or is bedridden. Flexible straws, and cups with specially designed handles and spouts, enable a person to drink safely, without help.

Using a cup with a spout

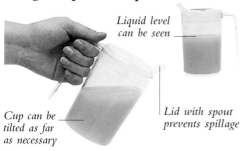

Liquid level can be seen

Cup can be tilted as far as necessary

Lid with spout prevents spillage

Using a hand-rest cup

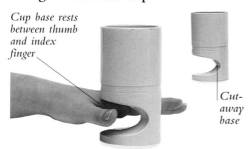

Cup base rests between thumb and index finger

Cut-away base

Using a two-handled cup

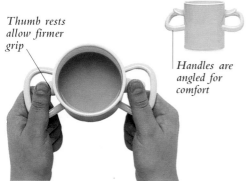

Thumb rests allow firmer grip

Handles are angled for comfort

EATING AIDS

Cutlery Specially shaped and thick-handled cutlery is designed for someone with a weak grip or someone who only has the use of one hand.

Knife/fork combination

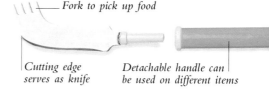

Fork to pick up food

Cutting edge serves as knife

Detachable handle can be used on different items

Spoon/fork combination

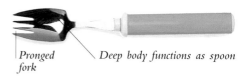

Pronged fork

Deep body functions as spoon

Angled spoon

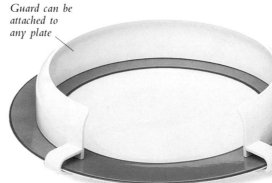

Angled head

Extra thick handle is easy to grip

Plate guard Someone who can use only one hand can get food on to a fork or spoon by pushing it against a plate guard.

Guard can be attached to any plate

MINOR DIGESTIVE PROBLEMS

IF YOUR RELATIVE IS ILL she may vomit, especially after eating. Steps should be taken to limit any distress this may cause and, if the problem persists, medical help should be sought. An immobile person may have difficulty digesting food, which can lead to a variety of uncomfortable symptoms, collectively known as indigestion; as a result her diet and eating habits may need to be changed.

WHY INDIGESTION CAN OCCUR

If your relative's indigestion is due to her inability to chew, provide soft foods and seek the advice of her GP. Indigestion may also be caused by the following:

◆ lying down or bending forwards after eating a large meal;

◆ eating spicy meals;

◆ eating too quickly;

◆ drinking too much alcohol, or drinking alcohol on an empty stomach;

◆ smoking.

Sites of discomfort

Heartburn is burning sensation in chest

Indigestion is discomfort in upper abdomen

VOMITING

This may be a sign of an underlying illness or infection, so check for other symptoms. If vomiting occurs often, pass the following information to the GP:

◆ the colour and content of the vomit (check in particular for any blood);

◆ whether vomiting is linked to eating and drinking;

◆ whether there is pain or diarrhoea.

To help, keep a bowl and flannel to hand and offer your relative the chance to freshen up afterwards.

EATING DISORDERS

Frequent vomiting can indicate eating disorders, such as anorexia nervosa or bulimia. Possible signs are:

◆ regular use of the lavatory after meals;

◆ avoiding meals altogether;

◆ losing a lot of weight.

Seek medical advice if you suspect these disorders.

INDIGESTION AND HEARTBURN

Indigestion usually occurs soon after eating or drinking. The symptoms can vary, but there is often a feeling of fullness and discomfort in the abdomen, perhaps accompanied by belching, nausea and heartburn. Your relative should take preventive measures to avoid it occurring.

Pinpoint the cause Try to work out why the indigestion is occurring (*see left*) and avoid the cause, if possible.

Neutralise stomach acid Sometimes the discomfort is relieved by milk or an over-the-counter antacid (ask the pharmacist to recommend one), but the GP should be consulted if the symptoms persist or recur.

CHAPTER 7

MAINTAINING &
IMPROVING MOBILITY

Your relative's ability to walk or move about may be impeded as the result of an illness or injury, or simply because he is frail; either way he will be more reliant on you for help. There are varying degrees of immobility, ranging from difficulty in getting out of a chair to the inability to stand up or walk. This chapter demonstrates the correct techniques for assisting your relative to move around the home, and illustrates the types of mobility aids that can encourage independence. An aid, such as a walking stick or walking frame, may enable your relative to undertake routine activities, such as shopping or visiting friends, by himself. This level of independence may greatly increase his confidence and assist in his recovery from illness.

TAKING CARE OF YOURSELF

There are strict guidelines for moving and handling an immobile person, which should be followed closely so that you avoid injuring yourself. If it is necessary for you to move your relative, ensure that the correct procedures are demonstrated to you by a healthcare professional, such as an occupational therapist, district nurse or physiotherapist. If your relative is very immobile, there are special aids and equipment available that are designed to make it safer and easier for you to move him.

HANDLING SOMEONE SAFELY

I F YOU ATTEMPT TO MOVE YOUR RELATIVE INCORRECTLY, you may injure yourself – particularly your back – or aggravate your relative's condition. These risks can be avoided if you follow the correct procedures for moving and handling a person. The techniques that are most appropriate for you and your relative should be demonstrated to you by a healthcare professional.

GETTING SPECIALIST HELP

If it is necessary to move your relative regularly, you must get specialist help. If you care for your relative on your own, it is especially important that you seek advice, as the risk of causing injury to yourself (particularly back strain), or to your relative, is increased.

Talking to a professional
The GP or district nurse can arrange for a specialist, such as a physiotherapist or an occupational therapist, to assess your situation and show you the correct procedures for moving your relative.

Using equipment If your relative needs a high level of assistance – if hc has to be helped into a bed or a bath regularly, for example – you should be shown how to use specialist equipment, such as a hoist (see page 92). You should also be shown how to maintain it.

PREPARING TO MOVE SOMEONE

If part of your relative's daily care involves moving him, always make sure that you are fully prepared for the task. (For guidelines on what you should do if your relative falls down, see pages 76–77).

The move Is there anyone who can help you to move your relative?

You Have you been shown how to carry out the move? Are you wearing anything unsuitable – such as high-heeled shoes – which may be dangerous?

Your relative Is your relative mobile enough to help with part of the procedure; is he able to move himself to the edge of a chair, for example?

Safety Have you got enough space to carry out the procedure safely? Are you attempting any procedures that have not been fully explained to you?

SAFETY GUIDELINES

Back strain is one of the most common injuries sustained in the process of moving a person. To prevent this, try to get someone else to help you, and make sure that you:

♦ do not move a person if you have a back injury;

♦ only move him if it is absolutely necessary;

♦ reassure the person and tell him what you plan to do;

♦ explain the task to any helpers and elect one person to give clear instructions;

♦ employ the proper techniques that will allow you to use your legs and body weight to provide the power for the move, and so avoid straining your back or arms;

♦ straighten your back when moving the person, and bend your knees, where necessary;

♦ only use equipment or moving and handling aids if their use has been fully demonstrated to you.

WAYS OF ASSISTING MOBILITY

T HE FOLLOWING PAGES SHOW YOU what you can do to help your relative if he has mobility problems. None of the techniques involve *lifting* but, instead, show you how to move your relative by transference of body weight. If he has been prescribed a mobility aid, encourage him to use it. Procedures for moving your relative in bed are covered in *Bed Comfort* (*see pages 83–96*).

HELPING SOMEONE TO WALK

Position yourself on the person's weaker side. Support him round the waist with one hand, preferably by grasping his belt or waistband, and hold the hand closest to you. This position will enable you to support him if he becomes unsteady (*see overleaf*).

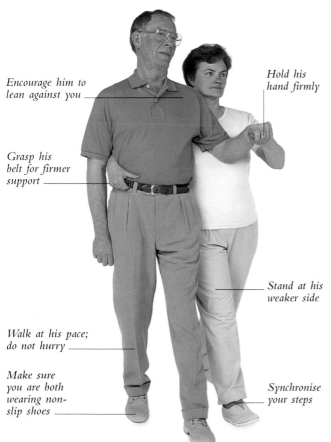

Encourage him to
lean against you

Grasp his
belt for firmer
support

Walk at his pace;
do not hurry

Make sure
you are both
wearing non-
slip shoes

Hold his
hand firmly

Stand at his
weaker side

Synchronise
your steps

CAUSES OF IMMOBILITY

Various conditions can cause immobility. (*See also* Glossary, *pages 178–80*).

Joint and bone problems Arthritis and rheumatism, and sprained or fractured limbs, will cause restricted mobility.

Convalescence Those who are weak after an operation or illness may need help to walk.

Conditions of the nervous system The nervous system, which controls movement, is affected by illnesses such as Parkinson's disease and multiple sclerosis.

Heart or breathing complaints Shortness of breath can restrict mobility (*see page 130*).

Stroke One side of the body may be paralysed, due to damage to the brain and nervous system.

Impaired vision Confidence to move about may be affected.

CONTROLLING A FALL

If you are helping your relative to walk and you think he is about to fall over, you can control his fall by using the method below, which involves slow and controlled movements that minimise the risk of injury to you and your relative. Never try to break a fall by catching the person or pulling him over to a seat.

Grasp both of his wrists as he falls

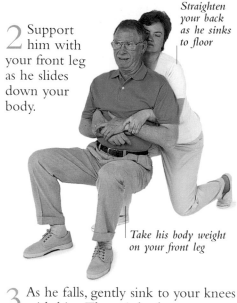

2 Support him with your front leg as he slides down your body.

Straighten your back as he sinks to floor

Take his body weight on your front leg

3 As he falls, gently sink to your knees with him. Then sit back on your heels for better balance, and support his head against your body.

Support him as you both sink to floor

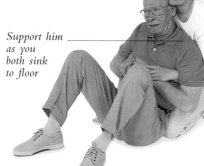

Get behind him as quickly as possible

1 Move behind the person. Grasp his wrists and fold his arms across his chest. With one foot in front of the other, lean into him and allow his weight to fall against your body.

MOVING SOMEONE FROM A WHEELCHAIR INTO A CAR

Open the car door wide and move the passenger seat back. Remove the side of the wheelchair nearest to the car and the footrest. Position the wheelchair as close to the car as possible, at a slight angle. Put the wheelchair brakes on. Using the same technique as you would to help someone out of a chair (*see opposite* and *page 78*), stand the person up and pivot him round so that the backs of his legs are against the car. Protect his head from hitting the top of the door frame as you lower him into the car, then gently swing his legs round into the car and make him comfortable.

HELPING SOMEONE
OUT OF A CHAIR

If your relative has problems getting up from a chair, it is advisable to invest in a chair with a high seat and firm armrests. The method below can also be carried out using a lifting sling (*see page 78*).

1 Help the person to move to the edge of the chair. Stand with your knees on either side of his and keep your back straight.

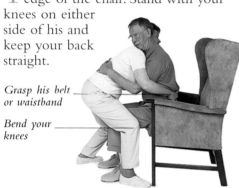

Grasp his belt or waistband

Bend your knees

2 Grasp his belt or waistband. Ask him to place his hands round your waist and to rest his head on your shoulder.

3 Begin with a rocking motion and bring your relative up with you on the count of three.

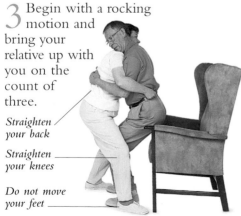

Straighten your back

Straighten your knees

Do not move your feet

4 Make sure he is steady and that you are both balanced before you release him.

ASSISTING SOMEONE
UP AND DOWN STAIRS

Use the procedures shown below to help your relative up and down stairs. Alternatively, consider installing an extra banister or stairlift (*see page 47*).

WALKING UP STAIRS
Stand two steps below the person. Ask her to hold on to the banister, and keep her steady by putting one hand on each hip. Walk up slowly.

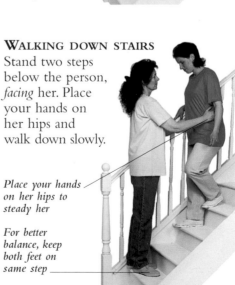

Climb stairs at her pace

WALKING DOWN STAIRS
Stand two steps below the person, *facing* her. Place your hands on her hips and walk down slowly.

Place your hands on her hips to steady her

For better balance, keep both feet on same step

ASSISTING SOMEONE WHO HAS IMPAIRED VISION

Before you offer to guide a visually impaired person, ask her if she would like your help. If you do not know each other, introduce yourself and ask her where she would like to go.
Method There are two ways to guide the person: either cup your hand under her elbow, or allow her to take your arm; if you are using the latter method, keep your forearm straight and steady. If possible, walk at her side; if not, walk a little ahead, but close enough to maintain contact. Do warn her of hazards at head height, and of any changes in ground surface. Tell her when you arrive at the destination and when you are about to leave.

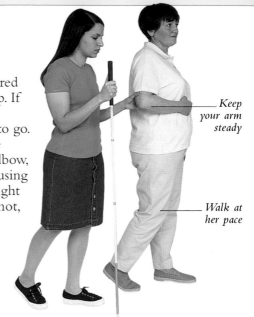

Keep your arm steady

Walk at her pace

HELPING SOMEONE WHO HAS FALLEN

If your relative falls, first deal with any injury and shock (*see pages 147–62*) and, if necessary, call an ambulance. If she is able to move by herself, follow the procedure described opposite to help her back on to her feet. If she is unable to move by herself, do not attempt to move her by yourself. If she is in immediate danger, having, for example, fallen close to water or to a heat source, you may have to move her, but try to get someone to help you.

FOR SOMEONE UNABLE TO MOVE

If your relative falls and is injured, call an ambulance. If she is uninjured, but unable to move, do not try to move her on your own. You can use a hoist if you have one (*see page 92*), but only if you have been trained to do so. If not, call an ambulance. Make her comfortable while you are waiting for help.

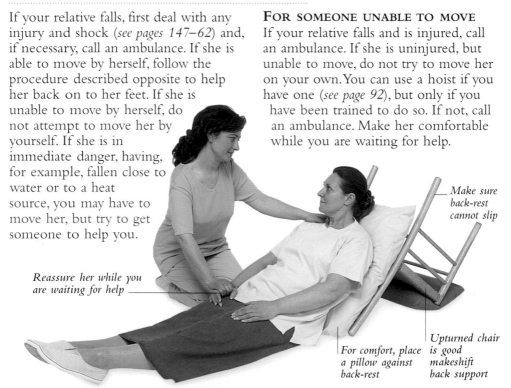

Reassure her while you are waiting for help

Make sure back-rest cannot slip

For comfort, place a pillow against back-rest

Upturned chair is good makeshift back support

FOR SOMEONE ABLE TO MOVE

If your relative falls, but is able to move, you can use the method shown below to help him pull himself into an upright position. This method requires two pieces of sturdy furniture of different heights, for example a low stool or a bedside table and an armchair. Place these as close as possible to your relative so that he can support himself and is not in danger of falling again.

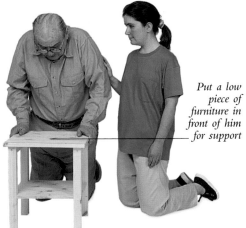

Put a low piece of furniture in front of him for support

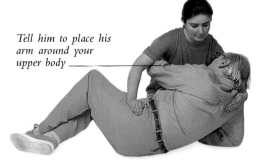

Tell him to place his arm around your upper body

1 Kneel next to the person. Place one hand on his uppermost hip and the other on his shoulder blade. Ask him to grasp you round the upper body.

3 Put a low, sturdy table in front of him and ask him to raise himself to a kneeling position by pushing down on the top of the table. Encourage him to use the table to steady himself.

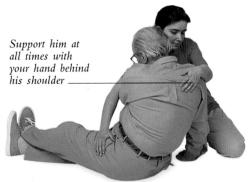

Support him at all times with your hand behind his shoulder

2 Using a rocking motion, on a count of three, press down on his hip and lean back on to your heels. This will assist him to a sitting position.

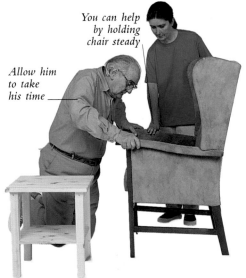

You can help by holding chair steady

Allow him to take his time

4 Place a chair next to the table. Ask him to let go of the table and grasp the arms of the chair. He should now be able to pull himself upright.

MOBILITY AIDS

THERE IS A WIDE VARIETY of equipment available to aid mobility. A healthcare professional, such as a physiotherapist, will know what is available and be able to advise you on the most suitable items for your relative. You may be able to borrow items from a charity organisation, local authority or health trust, or you may qualify for a grant (*see pages 164–68*).

MOVING AND HANDLING AIDS

The aids shown below make difficult tasks, such as helping someone out of a wheelchair or bed, easier and safer. The products are designed to give you greater control when moving someone, thus minimising the risk of injuring your back or arms. You should, however, only use these items if you have received proper instruction from a healthcare professional.

Turning disc This is useful for turning your relative round when you help him to move from a car into a wheelchair, for example. It works on the principle of one disc rotating over another.

Rubber, non-slip surface prevents person slipping

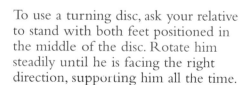

To use a turning disc, ask your relative to stand with both feet positioned in the middle of the disc. Rotate him steadily until he is facing the right direction, supporting him all the time.

Walk around with your relative as you rotate him

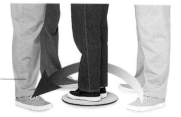

Lifting aids A lifting strap or sling is used to help someone up from a chair or to sit up in bed. The aid is placed round the person's waist if he is in a chair, or behind his shoulders if he is in bed. To help someone out of a chair, see page 75; to help someone sit up in bed, see page 88.

Lifting strap

Velcro fastening

Lifting sling

Hand grips

Using a lifting strap

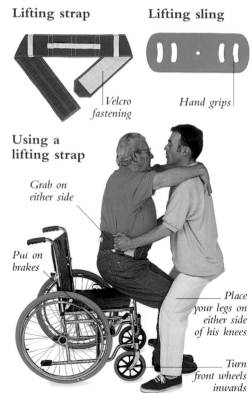

Grab on either side

Put on brakes

Place your legs on either side of his knees

Turn front wheels inwards

WALKING AIDS

The type of aid prescribed will depend on your relative's level of mobility. Sticks provide the minimum support, and frames the maximum. If he has an aid, encourage him to use it whenever possible; this will help him to get used to it and promote independence.

Walking sticks To be the correct height, the curve of the stick should be level with the crease of the wrist when the arm is straight. The person should wear his everyday shoes when it is measured.

Using a walking stick

If stick correctly measured, arm should slightly bend to grip it

Crutches These offer stronger support than walking sticks and may be used singly or in pairs. They should be correctly fitted and the person should be shown how to use them.

Using a crutch

Ensure handgrips are secure

Height can be adjusted

Non-slip rubber tip

Walking frames These are available without wheels or with two front wheels. The frame provides firm support, as the user can lean into it and grip it with both hands.

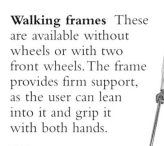

Using a walking frame

Lightweight aluminium frame

One with wheels is ideal if person cannot lift frame

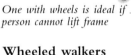

Wheeled walkers These give support to an immobile person while allowing him to carry out tasks such as shopping. Some walkers can also be folded flat.

Using a wheeled walker

Hand-operated brake

Basket for shopping

Four wheels make it easy to move

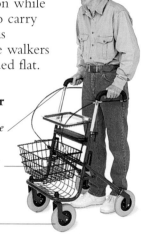

FITTING A WALKING AID

To ensure that walking aids are the correct height for the person using them, they should be measured and fitted by a physiotherapist or other trained person. If your relative is having difficulty using an aid, or it is causing discomfort, seek advice from a healthcare professional.

WHEELCHAIRS

THERE ARE SEVERAL DIFFERENT models of wheelchair available; the type recommended will depend on your relative's disability. In most cases, your local health authority will advise you and may even provide one. There are also independent organisations and charities who lend wheelchairs for short periods and arrange grants.

CHOOSING A WHEELCHAIR

There are two main types of wheelchair available.

Manual wheelchairs The rider-propelled model has large rear wheels so that the user can push himself along; transit chairs have small rear wheels so need to be pushed. Lightweight fold-up chairs are also available.

Powered wheelchairs These are used outdoors, indoors and for long distances.

WHEELCHAIR SAFETY

To ensure your own safety and the safety of your relative, follow these guidelines:
◆ never attempt to lift the chair alone with someone in it;

◆ if the chair has a seat belt, make sure it is securely fastened when the chair is in use;

◆ do not push a wheelchair forwards down a step or kerb if the person in the chair is at all heavy (*see opposite*);

◆ check brakes and tyre pressures regularly;

◆ make sure that the user is dressed safely and comfortably (*see page 106*).

Standard self-propelled wheelchair

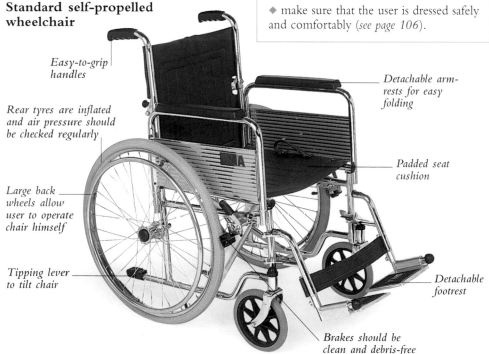

Easy-to-grip handles

Detachable arm-rests for easy folding

Rear tyres are inflated and air pressure should be checked regularly

Padded seat cushion

Large back wheels allow user to operate chair himself

Tipping lever to tilt chair

Detachable footrest

Brakes should be clean and debris-free

MOVING A WHEELCHAIR

When moving a wheelchair up or down a step or kerb, take your time so that the manoeuvre is safe. When tilting the chair, use the tipping lever.

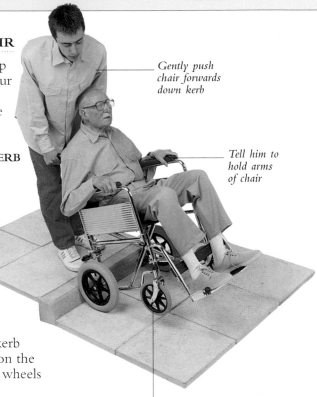

Gently push chair forwards down kerb

Tell him to hold arms of chair

GOING DOWN A STEP OR KERB

1 Face the step when approaching it. Tilt the wheelchair back by pushing down on the tipping lever with your foot.

2 With the chair tilted, push the back wheels to the edge of the kerb.

3 Push the chair down the kerb until the back wheels are on the ground. Then, lower the front wheels gently on to the ground.

Keep chair tilted until back wheels are on ground

FOR A HEAVIER PERSON

There is a danger that a heavy occupant may fall out of the wheelchair if it is facing forwards when you push it down. You should, therefore, reverse the position and lower the chair backwards. For this manoeuvre, do not use the tipping lever to tilt the chair.

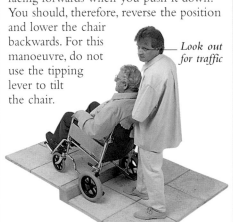

Look out for traffic

GOING UP A STEP OR KERB

1 Face the step when approaching it. Hold the handles securely. Place your foot on the tipping lever to tilt the chair backwards.

2 With the wheelchair balanced on its rear wheels, push it forwards until the front wheels are resting on the pavement or on the upper level of the next step.

3 Use your body weight to push the wheelchair forwards and up the step until the back wheels are on the same level as the front. *Never* attempt to lift the wheelchair.

COMPLICATIONS OF IMMOBILITY

PROLONGED IMMOBILITY may adversely affect your relative's physical or mental health. As a carer, you need to be aware of the likely consequences, and know how to help prevent or alleviate them. Because debilitating conditions may lead to boredom, anger, depression and isolation, you will also need to provide emotional support and encourage recreational activities (*see page 124*).

ENCOURAGING MOBILITY

Even if a person has mobility problems, he should be encouraged to undertake some form of exercise to minimise the risk of any complications occurring (*see right*). If your relative is confined to a wheelchair, seek advice from a healthcare professional about exercises designed specifically for wheelchair users.

Encouraging gentle exercise Your relative should be encouraged to:
◆ undertake gentle exercise, such as short walks or swimming in a warm pool; these activities will help to improve his circulation;

◆ find out about local activities, such as sports or dancing, specifically arranged for people with disabilities;

◆ embark on or continue a hobby, such as gardening, that involves some form of exercise.

PHYSICAL EFFECTS OF IMMOBILITY

Immobility can sometimes lead to further complications, such as infections or poor circulation. It may be possible to minimise these complications by seeking the advice of the GP or district nurse and by following the suggestions below.

Urinary tract infections Sitting for long periods of time may prevent the bladder from emptying properly. Residual urine can stagnate in the bladder, which may result in infection. Encourage your relative to drink plenty of fluids to ensure urine flow.

Constipation Physical inactivity can lead to constipation (*see page 108*), but a high-fibre diet and plenty of fluids can help to minimise this. If the problem persists, seek medical advice.

Chest infections Lying down for long periods causes mucus to stagnate in the lowest part of the chest. Regular changes of position can help to displace the mucus, so helping to prevent infection.

Circulatory problems Poor circulation can result from long periods of physical inactivity. Gentle physiotherapy may be recommended, or your relative may be prescribed special support stockings. If he complains of any sudden pains in his lower limbs or chest, tell the GP or district nurse immediately.

Pressure sores If your relative's condition results in him lying or sitting in one position for long periods, he is at risk of developing pressure sores (*see page 96*). These occur in areas where skin and tissue are squeezed between the bones and an underlying surface; blood supply to the tissues is restricted so starving them of nutrients. To prevent pressure sores, an immobile person should change position (*see page 90*) about every two hours. If pressure sores develop, seek urgent medical treatment.

CHAPTER 8

BED COMFORT

Looking after someone who is confined to
bed can be tiring and time-consuming for you, and
frustrating and restrictive for the person affected. This chapter
illustrates several aids and techniques to help you
provide a bedridden person with the safest and
most effective care.

MOVING A PERSON IN BED

You may have to help your relative into and out
of bed, and even change her position once she is in bed. If
you undertake these procedures incorrectly, you are in
danger of injuring yourself and your relative. This chapter outlines
effective ways of moving a person in bed; the procedures should,
however, be demonstrated to you by a healthcare professional. If
any specialist equipment is recommended, it is essential that you
be shown how to use it correctly.

REST AND SLEEP

You can improve your relative's quality of life by making
sure that she is as comfortable as possible in bed. This chapter
illustrates bed aids, such as specialist pillows and mattresses, that are
particularly useful for those who have to undergo long periods of
bed-rest. It also recommends ways that you can minimise any
physical discomfort or environmental disturbances that may
prevent your relative getting essential rest and sleep.

BEDS AND BEDDING

LOOK AT WAYS THAT YOUR RELATIVE'S existing bed can be adapted for her comfort and for your safety and convenience, as purchasing a new one may be disruptive for her. If your relative is in bed for long periods, you will need to change the bedding more often than usual. Make sure you have enough bed linen to be able to do this.

SELECTING THE BEST BEDDING

Choose bed linen that is machine-washable, easy to dry and comfortable.

Cotton covers Bed linen that is 100% cotton or a cotton mix is best, as it is less likely to cause a person to perspire. It can also be washed at high temperatures, which is an important factor if the person has an infectious disease or is incontinent. You will find fitted sheets easier to put on and keep flat.

Duvets Ideally, your relative should have two duvets: one with a low tog rating (the amount of thermal insulation it provides) for the summer, and one with a heavier rating for the winter.

Incontinence bedding If you are caring for someone who is incontinent, it is advisable to obtain a mattress protector and/or a bed protector (*see page 113*).

ADAPTING AND POSITIONING THE BED

To be able to care for someone effectively, the bed needs to be at the right height, not too wide and positioned so that you can reach both sides easily.
Bed height The mattress should be high enough for you to tend to your relative without having to bend too low. You may wish to use raisers to elevate the bed (*see page 52*), but first seek professional advice.
Bed size It is easier to care for someone in a single bed so that you can reach her easily, without overstretching. If your relative prefers to sleep in a double bed, encourage her to lie on one side of it so that you can reach her more easily.
Position and location Position the bed away from the wall so that you can move around it easily. You may also need to relocate your relative's bedroom if she has difficulty climbing the stairs or so that she can get to the toilet more easily.

MAKING THE BED

When you need to change the sheets, encourage your relative to get out of bed. If she is not able to do this, use one of the methods shown opposite to make the bed. Whichever way you make the bed, bear in mind the following guidelines:
♦ remove all the bedding and replace it with clean linen, or transfer the top sheet to the bottom so that you only have to put on a clean top sheet;
♦ stretch the bottom sheet to the corners of the bed and smooth away any wrinkles; if left they could rub against the skin and cause pressure sores (*see page 96*);
♦ tuck the top sheet in loosely to allow free movement of the feet, which can help to prevent pressure sores;
♦ keep a receptacle close at hand for dirty linen.

CHANGING SHEETS FOR A BEDRIDDEN PERSON

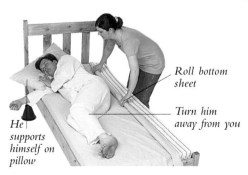

Roll bottom sheet

Turn him away from you

He supports himself on pillow

1 Roll up a clean sheet lengthways ready to use later. Turn the person on to his side (*see page 90*). Roll the soiled sheet up to his back.

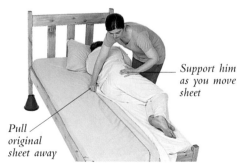

Support him as you move sheet

Pull original sheet away

3 Turn the person towards you over the two rolls and on to the clean sheet. Remove the soiled sheet and place it in a washing bag or basket.

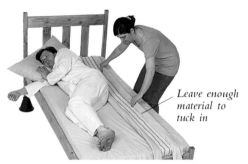

Leave enough material to tuck in

2 Place the rolled–up clean sheet on the edge of the bed, open end towards you. Unroll it to where the soiled sheet is placed.

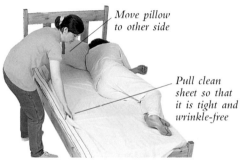

Move pillow to other side

Pull clean sheet so that it is tight and wrinkle-free

4 Unroll the remainder of the clean sheet across the bed and tuck it in. Then turn him on to his back again and make him comfortable.

FOR SOMEONE WHO CANNOT BE TURNED

If the person cannot lie on his side:
◆ sit him up (*see page 88*);
◆ roll the dirty sheet up to his back;
◆ replace it with a clean sheet;
◆ move him back up the bed on to the clean sheet (*see page 89*);
◆ remove the dirty sheet;
◆ pull the clean sheet from under his legs and tuck it in.

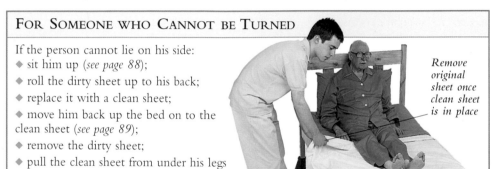

Remove original sheet once clean sheet is in place

AIDS TO COMFORT

IN ADDITION TO SUITABLE BEDDING, you may wish to buy one or two extra items that add to your relative's comfort in bed. Some of these aids prevent pressure sores, while others make activities, such as eating or reading in bed, easier and more enjoyable. An occupational therapist will be able to advise you on the choice of items that are most suitable for your relative's needs.

BED CRADLES

A bed cradle is placed under the mattress once the bottom sheet is on. The top bedclothes can then be draped over it to keep the weight of them off the person and prevent pressure sores.

MATTRESSES

Variable pressure mattresses can be made of spongy material or made up of a series of air pockets that inflate and deflate at different times. Both help to distribute the person's weight evenly so that the points at which the body comes into contact with the mattress are varied, thus helping to prevent pressure sores.

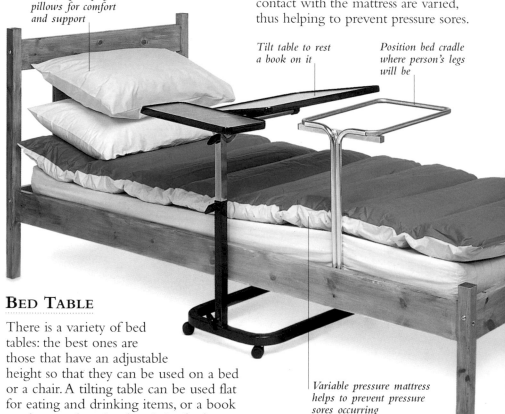

Provide plenty of pillows for comfort and support

Tilt table to rest a book on it

Position bed cradle where person's legs will be

BED TABLE

There is a variety of bed tables: the best ones are those that have an adjustable height so that they can be used on a bed or a chair. A tilting table can be used flat for eating and drinking items, or a book can be rested on it when it is tilted.

Variable pressure mattress helps to prevent pressure sores occurring

SUPPORTS

If your relative is confined to bed, it is essential that she sits up for some of the time. This is particularly important to prevent the onset of breathing difficulties and chest infections (*see page 82*). To enable her to sit up, she must have adequate pillow support. Provide plenty of normal pillows, placing them under her head, neck, shoulders and arms for support, and consider purchasing one of the specialist varieties shown below. For better support, the v-shaped pillow may need to be used in conjunction with ordinary pillows.

V-shaped support pillow

This is shaped to provide even support for the neck, back and arms.

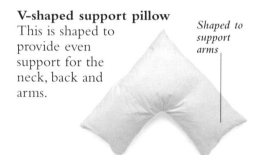

Shaped to support arms

Back support This armchair-shaped support is made from sculptured foam, and enables someone to sit up in bed.

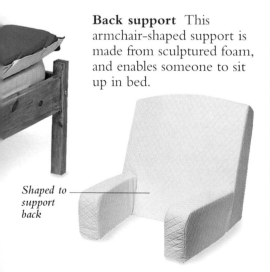

Shaped to support back

HOT-WATER BOTTLE

This provides warmth and comfort, and can help to minimise pain. The bottle should be covered with a fleecy cover to prevent burning.

Bottle and cover

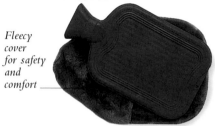

Fleecy cover for safety and comfort

HOW TO FILL A HOT-WATER BOTTLE

Lay the bottle on a flat surface. Holding the neck of the bottle steady, slowly pour in hot, but not boiling, water. Make sure no air pockets form: they can cause hot water to gurgle up and scald you. Fill the bottle ¾ full, gently push out any excess air and secure the cap. Wipe away any water and put the cover on.

SKIN PROTECTORS

These are made from towelling or fleecy fabric. They are designed for people who have to sit in a chair or lie in bed for long periods of time, to wear on areas of the body that are prone to pressure sores, such as the ankles, heels and elbows.

Ankle and heel protectors

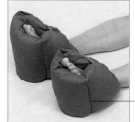

The ankles and heels are cushioned from the hard bed surface.

Velcro makes them easy to fasten

MOVING SOMEONE IN BED

THE TECHNIQUES FOR HELPING your relative into and out of bed, and for changing her position while she is in bed, should be demonstrated to you by a healthcare professional. The methods that you should be shown are outlined here. None of the techniques involve *lifting* but, instead, show you how to move a person by transference of body weight.

SAFETY GUIDELINES

Even if your relative is not heavy, *never* attempt to *lift* her from or in the bed as this may cause you to injure your back and arms. If you have not been shown the correct techniques for moving her, find someone to show you. Do not move someone by yourself if you can get help. Before beginning a move, always explain to your relative what you intend to do.

HELPING SOMEONE TO SIT UP IN BED

1 Face the person. Place one knee on the bed, level with her waist. Fold her arms across her chest. Slide a lifting sling (*see page 78*) under her shoulders. If you do not have one, use your hands instead.

Grasp handles of lifting sling

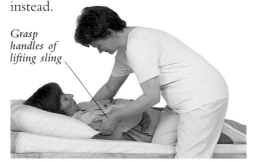

2 Using a rocking motion, lean back on to your heel on the count of three; this will transfer the person's body weight to you, bringing her upright.

Straighten your back

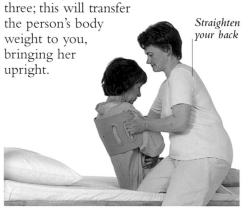

SITTING SOMEONE UP WITH HELP

Position yourself on the bed as shown above and ask your helper to do the same on the other side. Ask the person to fold her arms across her chest. Place one hand under her forearm and the other hand on her shoulder blade; ask your helper to do the same on the other side. Working together, use a rocking motion and lean back on your heels on the count of three to bring the person to a sitting position.

Place one hand on shoulder blade

Place one hand on arm

Her legs should be straight

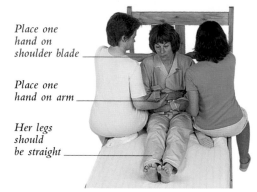

MOVING SOMEONE UP A BED ON YOUR OWN

You may need to move your relative up or down the bed so that you can change the sheets, for example (*see page 85*). The technique shown below allows you to use your body weight to power the move, so that you don't strain your arms and back. However, the technique is only effective if your relative is able to assist by pushing down on the bed with her feet.

1 Help the person to sit up (*see opposite*). Ask her to raise her knees.

2 Facing the same direction as her, place the knee nearest to her about 5cm (2in) behind her buttocks.

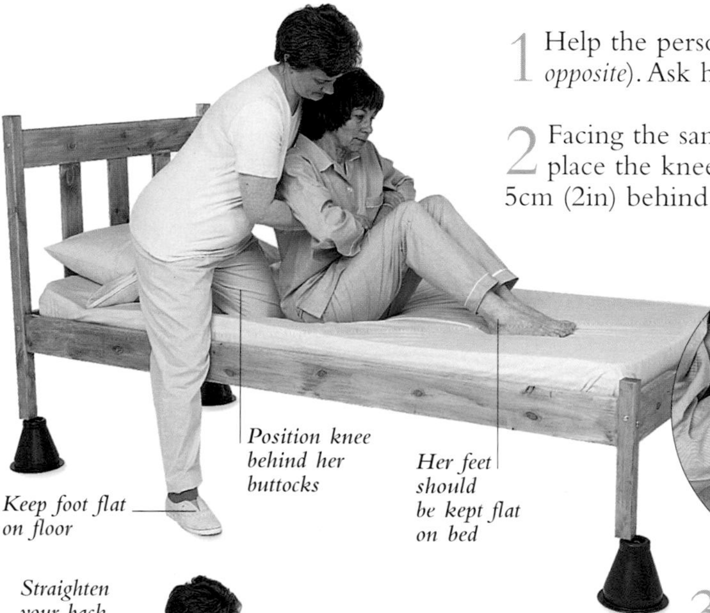

Position knee behind her buttocks

Her feet should be kept flat on bed

Keep foot flat on floor

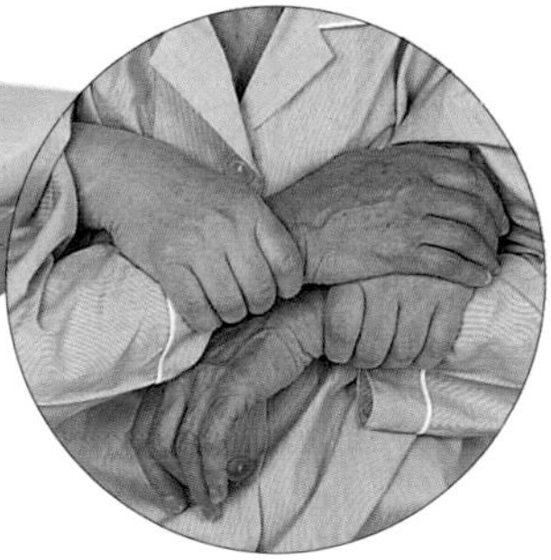

Straighten your back

Her legs straighten as you move back

3 Ask her to fold her arms across her chest. Reach under her arms and grasp her wrists gently, but firmly.

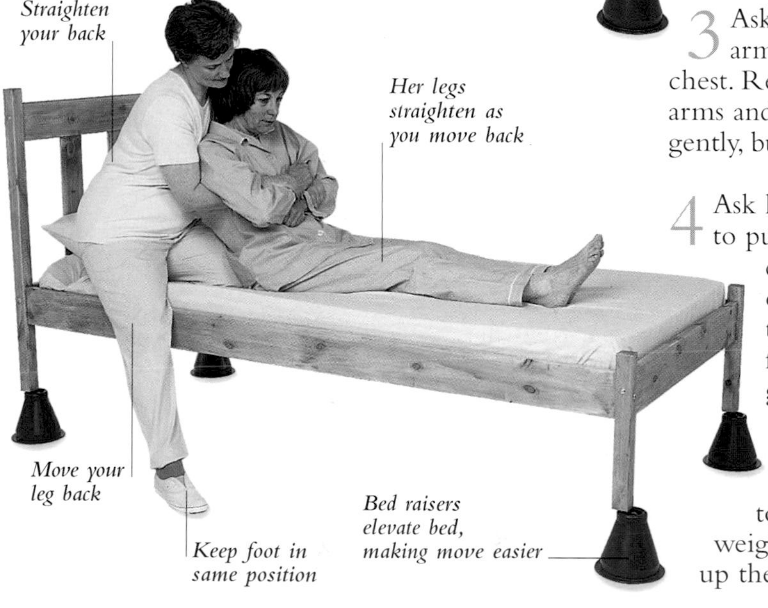

4 Ask her to get ready to push her feet down on the bed on the count of three. Keep your foot on the ground static and lean back on to the heel of your bent leg, to transfer her weight and bring her up the bed.

Move your leg back

Keep foot in same position

Bed raisers elevate bed, making move easier

CHANGING SOMEONE'S
POSITION IN BED

If your relative is confined to bed for long periods and cannot move herself, you will need to change her position approximately every two hours to prevent pressure sores developing. The procedure below shows you how to move your relative, with the aid of a helper, so that she can be turned on her side. Alternatively, you can obtain a sliding sheet (*see page 92*) that will enable you to move her by yourself.

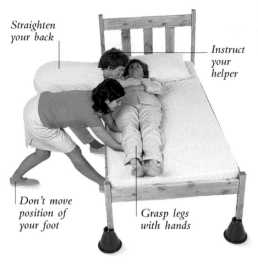

Straighten your back

Instruct your helper

Don't move position of your foot

Grasp legs with hands

1 Slide your hands, palms downwards, under the natural hollows of the person's upper body – the shoulders and small of the back. Ask your helper to slide her hands under the lower hollows – the thighs and knees.

3 On a count of three, both straighten your front legs and transfer your weight on to your back legs; the person will move across as you lean back.

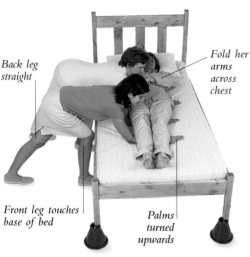

Back leg straight

Fold her arms across chest

Front leg touches base of bed

Palms turned upwards

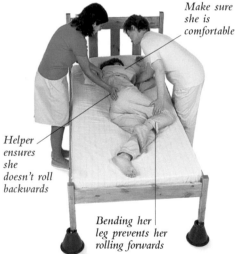

Make sure she is comfortable

Helper ensures she doesn't roll backwards

Bending her leg prevents her rolling forwards

2 Position yourself with one leg in front of the other, with your back leg straight and your front leg bent and touching the base of the bed. Turn your palms upwards. Ask your helper to mirror your position.

4 Grasp the person's far leg and shoulder to turn her on to her side. Ask your helper to support her from behind as she is turned. Let her make herself comfortable once she is lying on her side. Cover her with bedding.

Helping Someone to Get Out of Bed

Encourage your relative to get out of bed as often as possible, even if it is only to sit in a chair; it may be detrimental to her health to stay in bed for long periods. The method below can also be used if you want to move her to the edge of the bed to change her nightwear.

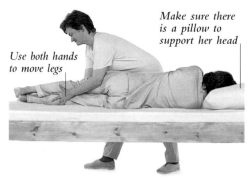

Make sure there is a pillow to support her head

Use both hands to move legs

1 Turn the person on to her side (*see opposite*). Stand beside the bed, level with her waist. Place your hands behind her knees and gently draw her legs out of the bed so that they dangle down towards the floor.

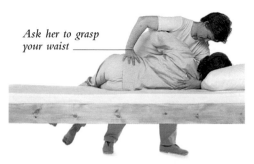

Ask her to grasp your waist

2 Ask her to place her upper arm around your waist; do not let her grasp you around your neck. Place one of your hands on her hip and the other hand on her shoulder blade.

Moving from a Bed

Once you have positioned your relative on the side of her bed, you may want to move her to a chair, wheelchair, commode or just help her to stand up. There are various ways you can do this, but, ideally, you should seek the advice of a healthcare professional – she should be able to advise you on equipment and the best technique for your relative's needs.

Helping her into a standing position Using the technique for getting someone out of a chair (*see page 75*), raise your relative to a standing position. Alternatively, to make the task easier, you could use a device such as a lifting sling (*see page 78*).

Helping her into a chair Once your relative is standing, help her to turn round and sit in the chair (or wheelchair or commode). Alternatively, use a turning disc (*see page 78*). The person stands on this and is gently swivelled round so that she is facing in the correct direction to be seated.

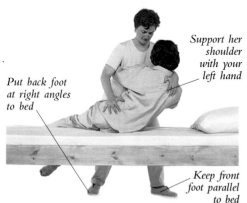

Support her shoulder with your left hand

Put back foot at right angles to bed

Keep front foot parallel to bed

3 Press down on her hip and lean back on to your back leg as you do this. This movement will bring the person to a sitting position. Make sure she is steady before you let go of her.

MOVING AND HANDLING AIDS

THERE IS A VARIETY OF AIDS that can be used to help a person who has restricted mobility in bed: some are designed to make the carer's task safer and easier, while others enable an immobile person to be more independent. It may be possible to borrow bed aids from a local authority or charity, which can be ideal if they are only needed for a short time.

AIDS THAT HELP A CARER MOVE SOMEONE

If your relative needs regular help to get into and out of bed, or you have to change her position in bed, you will probably be advised by an occupational therapist to obtain equipment to help move her. The way in which the equipment is operated and installed can vary, depending on the type used, especially for a device such as a hoist. Always ask for a demonstration and read the manufacturer's instructions before attempting to use any device.

Sliding sheet This is a piece of material, with a slippery surface, that allows you to move a person across the bed when she needs to be turned (*see page 90*). You slide it underneath her and, as you pull it towards you, she is automatically moved across with it.

Hoist This is an essential piece of equipment if your relative has to be moved regularly from a chair to a bed, or into a bath, for example. Most hoists involve sitting the person in a sling and, once she is securely in place, operating a winch system to lift her. A healthcare professional should be able to advise you on the hoist that is most suitable, and demonstrate how it should be used.

She is slowly moved into position

Press button to elevate hoist

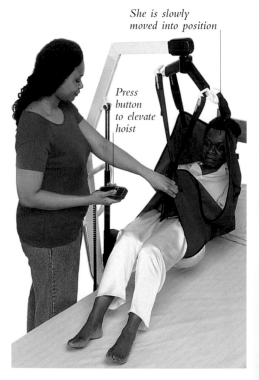

Place sheet underneath her

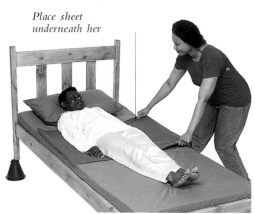

DEVICES THAT SOMEONE CAN USE UNAIDED

The aids shown here will help a person with some upper body strength to sit up and move around the bed without help.

Bed blocks These are "blocks" with handles that enable a person to move up and down a bed herself, or raise herself, on to a bed pan, for example. You can improvise bed blocks by tying two or three similar-sized books together.

Bed pole This is another device that can help a person with limited strength to sit up, adjust her position and get into and out of bed. It is suspended from a strong frame that sits under the head of the bed.

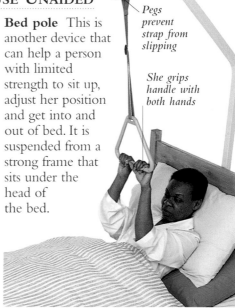

Pegs prevent strap from slipping

She grips handle with both hands

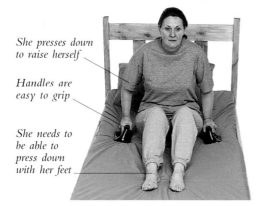

She presses down to raise herself

Handles are easy to grip

She needs to be able to press down with her feet

Rope ladder This device enables a person with reasonably strong hands and arms to raise himself to a sitting position. One end of the ladder is fastened to the bottom end of the bed; the user then pulls on the rungs.

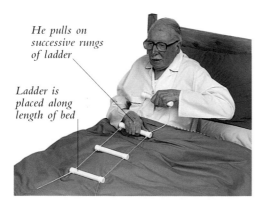

He pulls on successive rungs of ladder

Ladder is placed along length of bed

ADJUSTABLE BEDS

There are various mechanical beds that can be hand-operated to enable a person who has limited mobility to sit up, change position and get out of bed without help. Some types are fitted with a hand pump, others with an electric motor, that enable the person to adjust the head, back, knee and foot sections of the bed to the most suitable position.

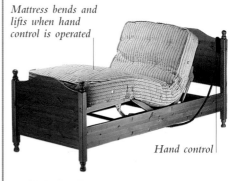

Mattress bends and lifts when hand control is operated

Hand control

Rest and Sleep

It is essential for your relative to get enough rest and sleep to restore energy, help the recovery process and improve morale. Get to know her sleep patterns and in times of wakefulness or restlessness, try to determine whether the cause is due to physical discomfort, anxiety or environmental disturbances. Sleeping pills should only be taken if prescribed by a doctor.

Physical and Psychological Discomfort

If your relative cannot get comfortable or relax, she may have difficulty sleeping. It is important that her bed is comfortable, that any pain or physical discomfort is minimised and that she is not kept awake by anxiety. Make sure she has everything that she needs to hand, night-time medication and a drink, for example; this may help to minimise the length of time that she is kept awake. She may also like a book so that she can read herself to sleep.

SOLVING PHYSICAL AND EMOTIONAL PROBLEMS		
PROBLEM	WHY IT OCCURS	SOLUTIONS
Hunger or thirst	If a person wakes in the middle of the night, hunger and thirst can prevent her getting back to sleep.	Make sure she has enough to eat and drink during the day. Place a drink and snack on her bedside table at night.
Physical discomfort	The bed or bedding itself may be uncomfortable and aggravate physical problems. Wakefulness may also be caused by physical discomfort such as aching limbs, stiff joints or a full bladder.	Make your relative comfortable in bed. Check that bedding is not too heavy, sheets are not wrinkled or wet and pillows are a comfortable height. An immobile person should be provided with a toilet aid, such as a commode (see page 114).
Pain	Pain in the middle of the night may cause psychological as well as physical discomfort.	Make sure that she has taken the correct dosage of pain-relief medicine and that any painkillers required are to hand.
Anxiety	A person may be kept awake because she is depressed or worried about her illness or a forthcoming operation.	Encourage your relative to talk about her concerns. Find ways for her to relax before bedtime, such as reading.

Environmental

Disturbances

A change of environment may cause your relative to feel very disorientated, which can have a disruptive effect on sleep patterns. To minimise this, try to keep her bedtime routine as familiar as possible. If you have very noisy neighbours, explain to them that your relative needs to rest; you will find that most people will be sympathetic. It may also be worthwhile purchasing earplugs for your relative – they are available from chemists – especially if she likes to sleep during the day or goes to bed early.

Sleep Patterns

Your relative should not become overtired, as this may hinder her recovery. Try to keep to her natural pattern of sleeping, and encourage her to follow this as closely as possible. If she is prevented from taking a customary nap in the afternoon, for example, she may want to sleep in the evening, which may then make it difficult for her to sleep during the night. Make sure that you are not deprived of sleep as well. If you get very tired, try to adapt your own sleep patterns around those of your relative: when she sleeps, use the opportunity to rest yourself.

Minimising Environmental Disturbances

Problem	Why it Occurs	Solutions
Light	The room is too light or too dark at night.	If it is too dark, open the curtains or leave a light on. If it is too light, put up thicker curtains or line existing ones.
Odours	If the room has an intrusive smell it can disturb sleep.	Leave a window or door ajar so air can circulate. Use potpourri or flowers to freshen the room.
Change of environment	Your relative is not in her usual room, or has been relocated to a different building altogether.	If your relative is staying elsewhere, ensure that the rest of her bedtime routine remains as undisturbed as possible to minimise any disruption caused.
Room temperature	Your relative is too hot or too cold at night.	Open or close windows and adjust heating and bedding as necessary; check her temperature (see page 128).
Noise	Noises outside and inside the house can disturb normal sleep patterns.	Try to remove the source of the noise; failing that, "soundproof" the room by stuffing a rolled-up sheet or towel along the gap under the door.

PRESSURE SORES

WHEN SOMEONE HAS TO SPEND long periods of time in a bed or chair, she may be vulnerable to developing pressure sores. These sores occur in areas where the skin and underlying tissue are compressed between a surface and the bone, cutting off the blood supply to the affected area. Taking simple precautions can minimise the likelihood of pressure sores developing.

PREVENTING PRESSURE SORES

The following steps can help to prevent sores developing:

◆ encourage the person to get out of bed as much as possible;

◆ encourage her to move regularly. If she has very limited mobility, you will need to change her position every two hours (*see page 90*);

◆ always move the person in the proper way (*see pages 88–89*); do not drag her limbs up or down the bed;

◆ never allow her to lie or sit in wet or damp conditions;

◆ make sure the bedding is not irritating the skin and wash the bedclothes regularly;

◆ ensure that she is eating a balanced diet (*see page 61*);

◆ inform the GP or district nurse about any skin changes, such as redness, dryness or cracking.

VULNERABLE AREAS

If your relative is weak or unconscious, and therefore unable to move in bed, there is a risk of pressure sores developing. These occur in places where the bones are very near the surface of the skin. The weight of the body reduces the blood supply to the skin tissues, causing the skin to change colour, initially to a pinky red. Areas that are vulnerable include:

◆ the head;

◆ the shoulders;

◆ the elbows;

◆ the base of the spine;

◆ the hips;

◆ the heels and ankles.

CAUSES OF PRESSURE SORES

Your relative may be vulnerable to pressures sores if:

◆ she remains in one position for too long;

◆ she has lost a lot of weight through illness, and therefore has less body fat to cushion the bones;

◆ there is friction on the skin, caused by the top sheet being too tight or by her being dragged across the bed, especially if her skin is not clean and dry.

WHAT ACTION YOU SHOULD TAKE

Pressure sores require swift medical attention. If you notice an area that is red, or one that appears blistered and tender, for over 24 hours, inform a healthcare professional, who will assess and determine what treatment is required. If the skin has broken, the sore is more prone to infection and may take longer to heal. As well as treating the sores, the GP or district nurse may suggest the use of pressure-relieving aids (*see pages 86–87*).

CHAPTER 9

PERSONAL CARE

It is essential to your relative's self-esteem and self-respect that she is able to maintain a good standard of personal hygiene and dress herself. This will help to make her feel better about herself and to cope more positively with her condition.

ENCOURAGING INDEPENDENCE

Your support and encouragement are essential, especially if she is relearning basic skills that she once took for granted, such as brushing her teeth or putting on socks and shoes. Encourage her to carry out as many of the tasks as she can on her own and resist the urge to help, even if she is taking a long time. She may benefit from using some of the aids shown in this chapter; an occupational therapist will be able to advise you on which items are most suitable.

HELPING YOUR RELATIVE

It may be necessary for you to help your relative to wash and dress. In this situation you need to find the safest and easiest ways to do this and, if necessary, seek advice from a healthcare professional, such as a district nurse or an occupational therapist. If your relative is confined to bed, you may be shown how to give a bedbath; if she has severe mobility problems and you do not have a shower cubicle, an occupational therapist may recommend the use of equipment to help you to move her into and out of the bath.

Helping Someone to Wash

Always encourage your relative to, at the very least, wash her hands and face at a basin by herself. If she has mobility problems or is weak, you may have to adapt the bathroom to enable her to use it by herself (*see page 50*). If it is necessary to help her into a bath, always seek advice about the safest way to do this; an adapted shower cubicle may be a safer option.

Helping Someone to Have a Shower

An immobile person who cannot climb into a bath should be encouraged to use a shower cubicle. If she has difficulty standing in the shower, obtain a shower seat (*see page 51*); if she is confined to a wheelchair, a chair can be obtained that can be wheeled into and out of the cubicle. It is also advisable to fit handrails and get a non-slip mat for the floor.

You can help your relative by:
◆ ensuring that she has all her toiletries;
◆ turning on the water and making sure it is the correct temperature;
◆ passing her the shower head once she is securely seated.
Leave her alone, unless she needs assistance and supervision throughout. Agree, beforehand, on a way for her to communicate that she has finished.

Helping Someone to Have a Bath

If your relative cannot climb into the bath by herself, you may have to help her. You must not, however, attempt to lift her into or out of the bath. Seek the advice of a healthcare professional, who may suggest the use of specialist equipment, such as a hoist (*see page 92*) or bath lift, to enable you to move her. If your relative's mobility is only slightly impaired – she is just generally weak, for example – she may benefit from the use of some simple aids.

Grab rails The person can hold on to these as she gets into and out of the bath.
Non-slip mat This is placed in the bottom of the bath to prevent the person slipping as she gets in and out, and while she is sitting in the bath.
Bath board This is placed across the bath, so that the person does not have to turn or stretch to reach items.
Bath seat This is placed in the bath so that the person does not have to lower or raise herself so far.

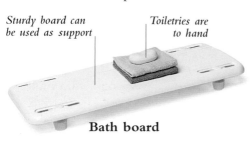

Sturdy board can be used as support   *Toiletries are to hand*

Bath board

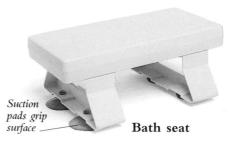

Suction pads grip surface

Bath seat

GIVING SOMEONE A BEDBATH

Your relative will require a bedbath if he is unable to get out of bed to wash. You will need a bowl of warm water, two or three towels, soap and two sponges or flannels; use different sponges for the face and genitals. Keep him warm by covering those parts of the body that are not being washed with a sheet and towel.

1 Remove the person's upper-body clothing. Pull the top sheet up to his armpits and cover it with a towel. Wash his face, neck, shoulders, arms and hands, and then dry these areas.

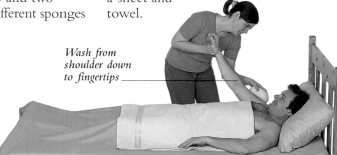

Wash from shoulder down to fingertips

2 Fold the sheet and towel down to his waist. Wash and dry his chest and abdomen; make sure that you dry thoroughly under any folds of skin as sores may develop in areas that remain damp or wet.

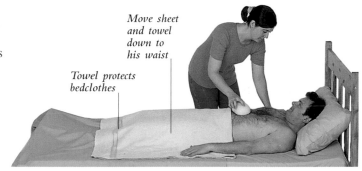

Move sheet and towel down to his waist

Towel protects bedclothes

3 Cover the top half of his body. Remove any lower-body clothing. Wash and dry his legs and feet. Allow him to wash the genital area himself with the second sponge. Cover him with the sheet, while you change the water.

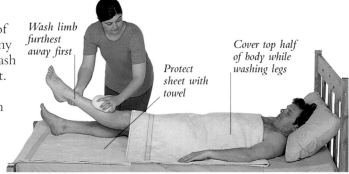

Wash limb furthest away first

Protect sheet with towel

Cover top half of body while washing legs

4 Turn the person on to his side (see page 90). Use the original sponge to wash his back and buttocks. Dry him and help him dress into clean clothes.

IF someone has difficulty lying on his side, sit him up (see page 88). Protect the bottom sheet with a towel and then wash and dry his back.

Washing Aids

Stiff joints, poor balance or a general lack of mobility may make it difficult for your relative to wash herself. To enable her to clean all parts of her body thoroughly, you can purchase specialist washing aids: the most useful features are long handles to minimise the amount of stretching required, and straps for those who have difficulty gripping.

Useful Items for Washing

Specially adapted washing aids are useful for those who have difficulty bending or stretching, and for those who cannot grip a normal sponge, brush or flannel. There are several items shown below. Most of these items can be obtained from a chemist; if what you need is not in stock, it may be possible to order it. Choose items that are easy to clean. If you are not sure which aids are the most suitable for the person in your care, seek advice from an occupational therapist, who is trained to assess individual requirements.

Flannel strap

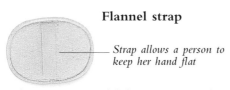

Strap allows a person to keep her hand flat

This item is useful for a person who cannot grip a flannel. She holds it by pushing her fingers under the strap.

Long-handled brush

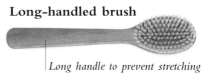

Long handle to prevent stretching

Sweeping along the arms and legs with this soft-bristled brush can slough dead skin and stimulate circulation.

Long-handled sponge

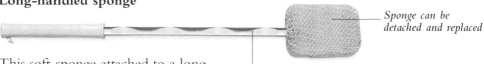

Sponge can be detached and replaced

This soft sponge attached to a long handle is designed to reach awkward areas such as the legs, feet and back.

Length of handle can be adjusted

Back strap

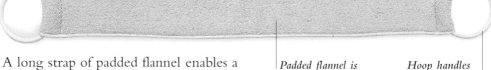

A long strap of padded flannel enables a person with limited mobility to wash parts of the body she finds difficult to reach.

Padded flannel is soft on skin

Hoop handles are easy to grip

CARE OF GENERAL APPEARANCE

A S WELL AS STAYING CLEAN, it may be important to your relative's self-esteem to look as presentable as possible – even if she is feeling unwell. Applying make-up does not have to be part of her daily routine if she does not want it to be, but when people are visiting, or when she is going out shopping or to the day centre, it may help to boost her confidence.

APPLYING MAKE-UP

You can obtain several useful items that can help your relative to apply make-up without your help.

Magnifying mirror A closer and clearer view can be achieved with a magnifying mirror propped up on a stand for easy use.

Foam tubing Specialist tubing can be attached to items such as lipsticks, eye pencils and mascaras, to make them easier to grip and thereby easier to apply.

Make-up bag Attach a long ring pull to the zip on a make-up bag, or replace the zip with velcro, so that someone who has difficulty gripping can open and close it easily.

Containers It may be better to purchase creams and lotions in pots, as a person with limited dexterity may find it difficult to squeeze a tube.

HELPING SOMEONE TO SHAVE

If you are caring for a man, you may need to help him shave. Always ask him whether he would prefer a wet shave or an electric shave. An electric razor may be easier for you to use if you are not practised or confident in the art of giving a wet shave. Always ensure that the equipment is clean.

GIVING A WET SHAVE

You will need a razor, shaving cream or soap, and water. Rub the soap or foam into a lather over the area to be shaved. The person may be able to do this himself. Then, hold the skin taut with one hand and firmly pull the razor down the cheek in long strokes. The razor should be sharp enough to cut the stubble and not scrub across his face. Rinse the razor after every few strokes. Rinse the face when you have finished.

USING AN ELECTRIC RAZOR

The hand-over-hand method gives some independence to a person who is able to grip an electric razor, but unable to rotate it. Once he is holding the razor, place your hand over his to direct it.

Using the hand-over-hand method

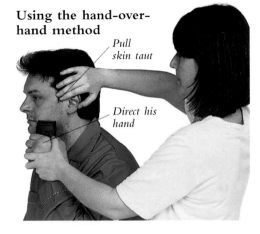

Pull skin taut

Direct his hand

CARING FOR THE HAIR

CLEAN AND GROOMED HAIR, even if it is just simply brushed to remove tangles and styled so that it is neat and manageable, may have a significant effect on how your relative feels about herself. A hairwash, especially, can be very refreshing and uplifting. Regular haircuts will make hair easier to manage – if your relative is housebound, find a hairdresser who can come to your home.

GENERAL HAIR CARE

Unless your relative is very weak, she should be encouraged to brush or comb her hair by herself.

Brushing hair If your relative's condition means that she has to lie or sit in the same position for long periods of time, her hair may become tangled. Lying on tangled hair may cause the scalp to become sore, possibly resulting in pressure sores (*see page 96*). To prevent this occurring, encourage your relative to brush or comb her hair gently, at least twice a day.

Wig care Your relative may have had treatment that has led to hair loss, such as chemotherapy (*see page 123*). If she wishes to wear a wig, consult a specialist for advice. Wash artificial wigs by hand; natural hair wigs should be washed and styled by a hairdresser.

WASHING THE HAIR

Having the hair washed can be very refreshing for someone who is ill. Your relative should wash her hair in the bath or shower, if possible. Ask the pharmacist for a dry shampoo or no-rinse shampoo so that she can keep her hair clean between washes.

For someone confined to bed If your relative cannot get up, you can obtain a device to wash her hair while she is lying in bed (*see right*). Alternatively, you can wash it by:
◆ laying plastic sheeting or towels over the bed and floor;
◆ positioning the person so that she is sitting up and leaning over a bowl on a bed table. If it is difficult for her to sit up, she can lie with her head over the bottom end of the bed, pillows under her neck and shoulders, and a bowl beneath her head.

HAIR WASHING TRAY

This inflatable tray allows a person to lie flat while his hair is being washed; it is especially useful for someone who has very limited mobility. Place a bowl beneath the hose to collect the water that drains from the tray.

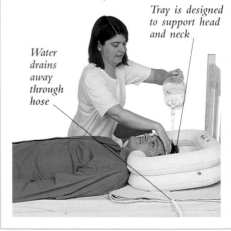

Tray is designed to support head and neck

Water drains away through hose

GENERAL BODY CARE

MEDICATION, SOME COURSES OF TREATMENT and general immobility may lead to uncomfortable physical side effects. Many of the more common complaints, such as mouth ulcers and eye infections, are treatable at home, as the chart below indicates. There may also be steps you can take to prevent the side effects occurring in the first place. Always seek medical advice, if necessary.

TREATING AND PREVENTING COMMON COMPLAINTS

AREA	COMMON COMPLAINTS	RECOMMENDED CARE
Mouth	◆ Cheek and gum ulcers caused by poor-fitting dentures. ◆ Lack of or excessive salivation, possibly as the result of a stroke. ◆ Poor oral hygiene, cold sores, dehydration and dry tongue.	◆ Consult a dentist about getting new dentures for your relative. ◆ Provide plenty of fluids and fresh fruit to encourage salivation. ◆ Encourage your relative to brush her teeth thoroughly and provide mouthwashes.
Eyes	◆ Difficulty blinking or closing the eyes as a result of a stroke. ◆ Eye infection.	◆ Wash around the eyes carefully. ◆ Drops or ointments may be prescribed to treat infection (*see page 135*).
Nose	◆ Blocked nose and sore nostrils from cold symptoms.	◆ Drops may be prescribed to relieve congestion (*see page 135*), or creams to soothe soreness.
Feet	◆ Corns, bunions and blisters. ◆ Fungal infections, such as athlete's foot. ◆ Pressure sores.	◆ Seek the advice of the GP for fungal infections, otherwise consult a chiropodist. ◆ Take steps to prevent pressure sores (*see page 96*) and seek medical advice.
Nails	◆ Hard, brittle nails, prone to splitting, on fingers and toes. ◆ Ingrowing toenails.	◆ Seek the advice of a chiropodist. ◆ Trim nails regularly, cutting straight across and not down into the corners.
Ears	◆ Excessive wax, which may be soft or hard. ◆ Sores on the edge of the ears.	◆ Drops may be prescribed (*see page 135*). ◆ Take steps to prevent pressure sores (*see page 96*) and seek medical advice.
Skin	◆ Red, sore skin in the armpits, groin or breast areas. ◆ Dry, flaky skin. ◆ Rash caused by allergy.	◆ Ensure skin in these areas is kept dry. Do not allow talcum powder to clog. ◆ Moisturise regularly. ◆ Seek medical advice – an emollient cream may be prescribed.

DRESSING TECHNIQUES

I F YOUR RELATIVE'S MOBILITY OR DEXTERITY is impaired, the simple tasks of dressing and undressing may be frustrating and exhausting. Losing the ability to dress oneself – to put on a shirt or pull on a sock – can deal a severe blow to a person's independence and dignity. Dressing aids are designed to enable a weak or immobile person to dress herself more easily.

DRESSING AIDS

Most dressing gadgets are designed with long handles to prevent someone with limited mobility having to bend when she is dressing or undressing herself, thereby minimising the risk of injuries sustained by falling or over-stretching. All the items shown here are inexpensive and easy to use. An occupational therapist will be able to advise you on the products that are most suited to your relative's needs.

Dressing stick The double wire hook at one end enables a person to pull on or push off clothing. This aid is useful for someone with weak limbs.

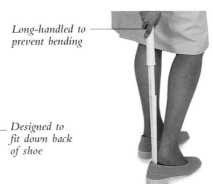

Long-handled shoe horn This enables a person to put on her shoes without having to bend, so minimising any risk of strain.

Long-handled to prevent bending

Designed to fit down back of shoe

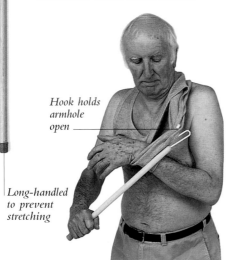

Hook holds armhole open

Long-handled to prevent stretching

Stocking aid The stocking is placed over the shaped plastic and then pulled up by pulling the straps.

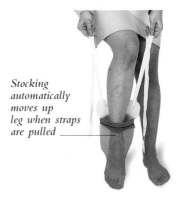

Stocking automatically moves up leg when straps are pulled

HELPING SOMEONE TO DRESS

Dressing and undressing can be a lengthy process for a weak or paralysed person. If possible, allow your relative to dress independently, but if he needs help, follow these guidelines:

◆ make sure he is sitting or lying down to make the task easier;

◆ dress the weak limb first;

◆ always place a garment over the arm before pulling it over the head;

◆ allow him to assist, if at all possible, but do not rush him.

HELPING TO PUT ON SOCKS

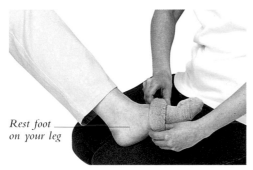

Rest foot on your leg

1 Fold over the top of the sock. Roll it back to halfway along the foot section and place it over the toes.

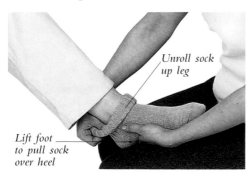

Unroll sock up leg

Lift foot to pull sock over heel

2 Supporting the underneath of the foot, unroll the sock over the foot, heel and up the leg.

DRESSING A PERSON WHO HAS AN INJURED ARM

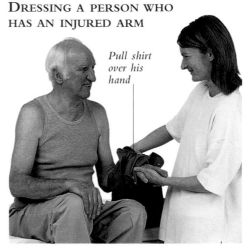

Pull shirt over his hand

1 Roll the sleeve down to the cuff. Place your hand through the cuff opening and take hold of the person's hand. Pull the shirt from your own hand over his.

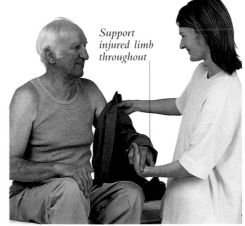

Support injured limb throughout

2 Keep hold of his hand and gently pull the shirt sleeve up his arm to the shoulder.

3 Take the garment around his back, so that he can reach the other sleeve with his good arm. He can then continue dressing by himself.

Choosing Clothes

IDEALLY, LET YOUR RELATIVE CHOOSE the clothes she would like to wear; if she relies on you to buy them for her, always opt for colours and fabrics that you know she likes. As well as buying items that are comfortable, consider what is practical: for example, if your relative has dexterity problems, do not buy garments with small buttons or back pockets.

Features to Look For

Choose items that may enable a person to dress without help. For example:
- slip-on shoes;
- v-necked jumper;
- sweatshirt or T-shirt;
- wrapover skirt;
- clip-on tie.

If your relative has dexterity problems or is weak, consider how easy she will find it to manipulate the fastenings on garments (*see right*).

For Wheelchair Users

People who are wheelchair bound often find that their waist and hips broaden; users of manual chairs find that their shoulder and upper arm muscles also get bigger. It may, therefore, be necessary for them to wear larger clothing. For safety and comfort, the following are advised:
- close-fitting sleeves and cuffs to avoid catching fabric in the wheels;
- longer-length skirts for a woman so that they fall easily over her knees when she is seated;
- short coats or jackets so that the person is not sitting on them; long coats can also get caught in the wheels;
- low-heeled, well-fitting shoes with non-slip soles, as these are less likely to slip off the footrests;
- short scarves that can be tied easily so that they don't get caught in the wheels.

Simple Fastenings

Press studs Press studs (*poppers*) are fastened by pressing together both halves. Use instead of buttons.

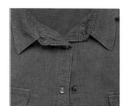

Large buttons Small buttons can be fiddly and difficult to grip. Choose garments with large buttons or replace small ones and widen the buttonholes.

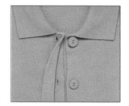

Drawstring waist Choose garments that have an elasticated waist. A drawstring is easy to tie and untie and an elasticated waist is more comfortable.

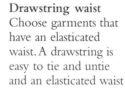

Velcro This consists of two nylon surfaces that stick to each other when pressed together. Replace buttons with velcro and resew them over the buttonholes.

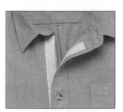

Invisible zip pull The catch is attached through the hole in the zip tag. The zip is moved by pulling the loop, which can then be tucked away.

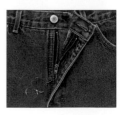

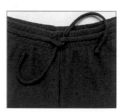

CHAPTER 10

BLADDER &
BOWEL CONTROL

Problems that affect the bladder and bowel range from
incontinence, constipation and diarrhoea, to abnormalities of the
urinary and lower digestive tracts.

INCONTINENCE

Looking after a person who has lost control of the
bladder or bowel – a condition known as incontinence – is
possibly one of the most difficult tasks for any carer. Incontinence
occurs when illness, injury or degeneration disturbs normal
bladder or bowel function, leading to the involuntary discharge of
urine or faeces. It is a distressing and embarrassing condition,
which may lead to the incontinent person isolating himself
and trying to cope alone. The problem must be addressed so that
ways can be found to allow the person independence and privacy
and so that, if possible, a medical solution can be found.

MEDICAL TREATMENTS

Medical advice should always be sought for bladder
and bowel problems. Solutions range from the prescription of
drugs, to treatment that diverts the passage of urine or faeces.
These treatments are now very refined and, with the proper care,
can significantly enhance the person's quality of life.

MINOR CONDITIONS

BLADDER AND BOWEL CONDITIONS, which include urinary problems, constipation and diarrhoea, may be the symptom of an underlying illness, an infection or a treatment. If your relative complains of any change in his bladder or bowel movements, such as discomfort or discolouration, or he has any difficulty in going to the toilet, you should always seek medical advice.

URINATION AND DEFECATION

Someone who is healthy will pass urine and faeces naturally.

How urine is passed:
◆ the bladder stores urine produced in the kidneys;
◆ as the bladder fills, nerve impulses signal to the brain that the bladder is full and must be emptied;
◆ the urine is passed – and discharged – through a tube (the *urethra*) connected to the bladder.

How faeces are passed:
◆ digestion takes place as food passes from the stomach to the small intestine;
◆ any nutrients are absorbed into the bloodstream; what remains passes into the large bowel;
◆ this waste matter (*faeces*), which is no longer required by the body, is stored in the large bowel before being expelled via the rectum.

RECOGNITION AND TREATMENTS

Once you recognise that there is a problem, you can identify possible causes and explore treatments.

WHAT TO DO FOR URINARY PROBLEMS

Your relative may have an infection if passing urine causes stinging and discomfort, or if the urine:
◆ is dark or cloudy in colour, or contains blood;
◆ has a particularly pungent smell;
◆ is being passed in small quantities frequently.
Seek medical help Your relative's GP may need to prescribe medication to treat the infection if it is the cause of the urinary problem.

WHAT TO DO FOR CONSTIPATION

This condition occurs when the person has failed to open his bowels as normal. There may be an obstruction, or the waste matter (*faeces*) may have become dry, making it difficult to pass.
Seek medical help A doctor may prescribe laxatives, suppositories or, in severe cases, an enema.
Encourage toilet use Encourage your relative to use the toilet regularly, even though he may be reluctant to do so because his bowel movements are painful.
Adapt the diet Make sure he eats a balanced diet (*see pages 61–63*) and drinks plenty of fluids.

WHAT TO DO FOR DIARRHOEA

When a person passes liquid faeces at frequent intervals, the condition is known as diarrhoea.
Seek medical help The advice of a GP should be sought, especially if the person is elderly or ill.
Adapt the diet Give your relative plenty of fluids, including water with a pinch of salt. Abstaining from food for 24 hours may also help to relieve diarrhoea.

INCONTINENCE

THIS CAN BE URINARY OR FAECAL, although the latter is rare. Incontinence is a medical condition, but a person who has toilet "accidents" may be diagnosed as incontinent because he cannot cope with the normal sequence of events involved in going to the toilet. If your relative is incontinent, consult a healthcare professional to find an effective way to manage and treat the problem.

CAUSES AND TREATMENTS

CAUSE	WHAT HAPPENS	TREATMENT
Enlarged prostate gland	◆ The enlarged prostate gland blocks the passage of urine. The bladder fills up and then involuntarily releases an overflow of urine.	◆ Insertion of a catheter. ◆ Surgery or other treatment to remove the prostate gland.
Weak muscle tone	◆ The muscles that control the passing of urine or faeces become weak so that urine (and, rarely, faeces) are passed involuntarily after coughing or mild exercise. This is stress incontinence.	◆ Pelvic floor exercises. ◆ Toilet routine. ◆ Surgery.
Infection	◆ Someone who has an infection may have a strong urge to urinate followed by an involuntary emptying of the bladder. Passing urine may be painful, causing a burning sensation.	◆ Medication to treat cause of infection. ◆ Sufficient fluid intake.
Damage to the nervous system	◆ If the nervous system is damaged, the person may be unable to recognise his need to use the toilet.	◆ Relearning control. ◆ Use of toilet aids. ◆ Insertion of a catheter.
Constipation	◆ Faeces become impacted in the rectum (see opposite); liquid faeces may seep out. In some cases, the resulting pressure on the bladder may lead to urinary incontinence.	◆ Drugs, such as laxatives. ◆ A high-fibre diet and sufficient fluids. ◆ Regular enemas, if condition persists.
Immobility and dementia	◆ For both conditions, a person may have normal bladder and bowel function, but be unable to get to the toilet in time, or need help once there. With dementia, he may also be unable to express his need to go to the toilet.	◆ Toilet routine. ◆ Use of toilet aids (with supervision for someone who has dementia).

PROMOTING CONTINENCE

I F YOUR RELATIVE cannot be treated medically (*see page 115*), he may have to rely on the use of aids (*see pages 112-14*). However, by pinpointing why the incontinence occurs, you may be able to establish a toilet routine and address any mental or physical problems that are causing the difficulties. This may help your relative to regain continence or, at least, alleviate the problem.

PINPOINTING AND SOLVING THE PROBLEM

The chart below is designed to help you to identify the cause of the problem and give you guidance on how to help your relative to be continent.

However, always seek the advice of a healthcare professional, such as the GP, district nurse or continence advisor, as soon as the problem begins.

HOW TO HELP AN INCONTINENT PERSON

PROBLEM	AIM	WHAT YOU CAN DO
A paralysed person He may be physically unable to recognise that he needs to use the toilet.	To recognise that urine or faeces need to be passed.	**Encourage toilet use** To establish a toilet routine, make sure that your relative goes to the toilet, or is taken there, every 2–3 hours. **Establish a pattern** Note times that the incontinence occurs and, if a pattern emerges, prompt him about half an hour before these times. **Use reminders** Set an alarm clock or kitchen timer to ring when he usually needs the toilet.
A person with dementia He may know when he needs the toilet, but be unable to express this need. **An immobile person** He may be unable to get to the toilet.	To know where the toilet is and be able to get there.	**Deal with confusion** Decorating or moving house may disorientate a confused person. Tell the person where the toilet is or put up signs until he is more confident of his whereabouts. **Think about location** Ensure that an immobile person's living and sleeping quarters are near to the toilet. If necessary, put up handrails to help him get there, and make sure the route is free of obstacles. If he is unable to go to the toilet by himself, take him every 2–3 hours or obtain an aid for occasional use (*see page 114*).
A physically impaired person He may have difficulty undoing his clothes.	To undo or remove necessary clothing easily.	**Provide practical clothes** Ensure that your relative wears clothes that are easy to remove; avoid small buttons or difficult fastenings (*see page 106*). Don't leave him in pyjamas all day; it may worsen the incontinence if he feels he is not trusted.

Getting Help

Only one out of every ten carers looking after an incontinent person asks for help. Do not be afraid to use the resources available to you, and do not hesitate to find out if you qualify for financial help.

Specialist advice

Ask the GP or district nurse to refer your relative to a continence adviser, who will be able to assess his needs and advise you both accordingly. Seek advice from specialist organisations, such as the Continence Foundation (*see page 176*).

Incontinence aids

There is a wide variety of incontinence aids (*see overleaf*) available that will make it easier for you and your relative to deal with the problem. For example, specialist bedding will reduce the amount of washing you have to do and add to your relative's comfort. Some aids, such as incontinence pads, may be provided free of charge; find out what is available and suitable from a continence adviser.

Laundry

Continual washing can add to the burden of caring for an incontinent person. Find out if your local authority offers a laundry service.

Financial

Find out if you are eligible for benefits to cover the expense associated with incontinence (*see pages 164–68*).

Adapting an Incontinent Person's Diet

In some cases, adapting your relative's diet and fluid intake can help to control incontinence.

Food A high-fibre diet can help to prevent constipation, which may be the cause of faecal incontinence.

Fluid Limiting drinks in the evening may help if the urinary incontinence tends to occur at night. Do not, however, try to deal with urinary incontinence by limiting fluid intake during the day. It is essential to your relative's health that he drinks sufficient fluids.

Coping Emotionally

Incontinence can be a very difficult problem to cope with and, sadly, it is one of the main reasons why people give up their caring role. The problem is aggravated when the person does not admit to the problem and tries to cover up accidents by hiding soiled clothes, or when he appears to be incontinent on purpose. Before you can begin to deal with the problem, whatever its cause, it is important for both of you to be honest about how you feel.

Your feelings It is very normal to feel angry and disgusted by having to deal with incontinence. If you are finding it difficult to cope, seek help (*see left*). Trying to cope alone will not be beneficial for either you or your relative.

Your relative's feelings It is very likely to be embarrassing and frustrating for your relative if he has to rely on you because he is unable to carry out these most basic of functions. Allow him as much privacy and independence as possible. Encourage him to talk about it and try to be understanding.

INCONTINENCE AIDS

THERE IS A RANGE OF AIDS to help with incontinence. Ask to see a continence adviser, who will be able to assess the extent of your relative's problem, taking his age and mental and physical condition into account. She will also be able to give you advice on the devices most likely to help your relative, and provide information on available grants and benefits.

ALARM CLOCK

An alarm clock is useful if your relative does not recognise his need to go to the toilet. To establish a routine, set the alarm to go off every 2–3 hours as a reminder that it is time to use the toilet.

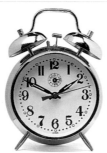

COMFORT AID

Commode ring This circular, air-filled ring is suitable for use on most commodes (*see page 114*). It is an aid to comfort and is especially useful if your relative is suffering from pressure sores (*see page 96*).

Commode

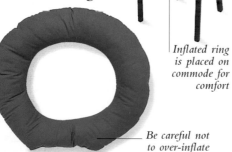

Commode ring

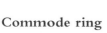

Inflated ring is placed on commode for comfort

Be careful not to over-inflate

PADS AND PANTS

Incontinence pads There are designs for men and women, and a variety of sizes and absorbency levels (double for maximum absorbency). They can be used with or without special pants. The pad, which works on the same principle as a nappy, will absorb moisture and ensure that the wearer's skin remains dry.

Male pad

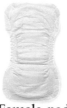

Female pad

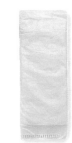

Double pad

Incontinence pants Special pants are available that have a pouch that holds an incontinence pad. The pad should be positioned well to the front for a man and further back for a woman. Encourage your relative to insert the pad himself, if he is capable. There are also washable, reusable pants that have a built-in pad.

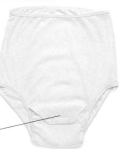

Waterproof pouch for pad

Bedding for an Incontinent Person

There is a wide variety of incontinence products available, from mattress and pillow protectors to incontinence sheets. There are different types of absorbency to suit the level of incontinence. You may not need all the items shown below; a continence adviser will recommend those most suitable for your relative. Where possible, choose bedding that is easy to wash and dry. A mattress protector may cause some people to sweat excessively; discontinue use if this happens. For your relative's comfort, and to prevent sores developing, always change wet bedding as quickly as possible.

Protecting bedding

1 Place a fitted water-proof protector over the mattress.

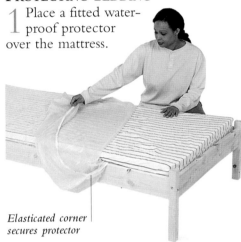

Elasticated corner secures protector

2 Put an ordinary bottom sheet on top of the protector and tuck it in securely.

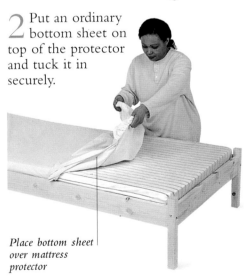

Place bottom sheet over mattress protector

Pillow protector *Pillowcase goes over protector*

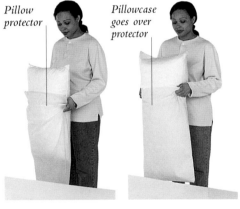

3 Strip the pillow of its cover and replace it with a waterproof protector. Put an ordinary pillowcase over the protector.

4 Place an absorbent bed protector over the bottom sheet.

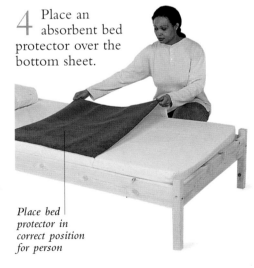

Place bed protector in correct position for person

TOILET AIDS

IF YOUR RELATIVE IS IMMOBILE OR BEDRIDDEN, he may benefit from the use of a toilet aid, such as a urinal, commode or bed pan. These aids will help to reduce the risk of him having an "accident", and give him a degree of independence when he is using the toilet.

USING SPECIAL TOILETS

When your relative wants to use a urinal, commode or bed pan, make sure:
◆ he is able to unbutton or remove the necessary clothing easily;
◆ there is a toilet roll to hand;
◆ he can be left in private, if possible.

After using the toilet, establish a way for your relative to communicate to you that he has finished, then:
◆ assist him to clean himself, if he is unable to do this on his own;
◆ ensure that he washes his hands;
◆ wash the equipment (see page 57);
◆ wash your hands (see page 56).

Urinals These are mainly used by men, but the pan type can be used by women, and is good for wheelchair use.
How to help Encourage your relative to use it alone, but if he is unable to do so, help him. It is difficult for a man to use a urinal lying down, so he may need to sit supported on the edge of the bed.

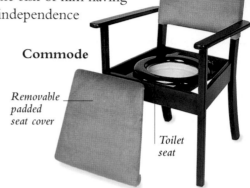

Commode

Removable padded seat cover

Toilet seat

Commodes These are chairs with a removable seat that conceals a built-in commode pan and toilet seat. Easy to clean, commodes are ideal for those who can get out of bed, but cannot get to the toilet.
How to help Help the person on to the commode, and give him as much privacy as his condition allows.

Bed pans These are used for a person who cannot get out of bed. The wedge-shaped slipper type is particularly easy to use, allowing the person to slide backwards and lift himself on to it.
How to help If it is a steel pan, make sure it is warm and dry. Ask him to raise himself, or help him to do this, then slide the bed pan underneath him. Provide a man with a urinal as well (see left).

Female urinal

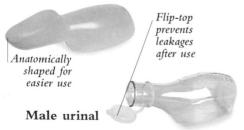

Anatomically shaped for easier use

Flip-top prevents leakages after use

Male urinal

Slipper bed pan

Wedge-shaped for easier positioning

MEDICAL TREATMENTS

I T MAY BE NECESSARY for a person with bladder and bowel problems to be fitted with a device that allows urine or faeces to be passed and collected through a different channel: a catheter for someone with urinary incontinence, or a stoma with a bag for someone with a disease of the digestive tract *(see overleaf)*. If properly maintained, these can enhance the person's quality of life.

CATHETER CARE

As part of the medical treatment for a bladder problem or as a last resort for untreatable incontinence, a tube (*catheter*) may be inserted into the bladder to drain urine. The tube is then attached to a collecting bag strapped to the person's leg or waist.

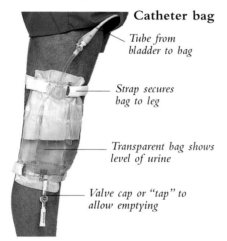

Catheter bag

Tube from bladder to bag

Strap secures bag to leg

Transparent bag shows level of urine

Valve cap or "tap" to allow emptying

LOOKING AFTER THE CATHETER

Most catheters are inserted into the bladder and left in place. The person will be shown when and how to empty the bag. The tube is replaced at varying intervals by a GP or district nurse. People with intermittent incontinence, such as those with multiple sclerosis, may be taught how to insert a catheter. To prevent infection, the person should wash the area around the catheter every day with soap and water, and drink plenty of fluids. You should understand the washing and emptying procedures, as you may have to assist your relative.

EMPTYING A CATHETER BAG

The bag should be emptied approximately every four hours or if it is more than two-thirds full.

Draining the bag The cap at the bottom of the bag is opened and the urine is drained into a container kept for this purpose. The urine is flushed down the toilet. If the bag is supplied separately, it may have to be changed. Follow instructions carefully and wear gloves to minimise the risk of infection.

Checking the tube After emptying, the tube that leads from the catheter to the bag should be checked to make sure it is not kinked or blocked.

DEALING WITH COMPLICATIONS

A catheter may cause a urinary infection. If your relative complains of a burning sensation when urinating and/or has cloudy urine, it may indicate an infection. Always seek medical help. If the catheter actually comes out, no attempt should be made to reinsert it as this may seriously damage the bladder or urethra. If complications arise, seek advice from a continence adviser or the GP.

STOMA CARE

When the digestive tract is diseased or damaged in some way, or it is not possible for the person to pass faeces normally, surgery may be necessary.

The stoma Part of the large intestine (a *colostomy*) or small intestine (an *ileostomy*) can be brought out on to the abdomen to form an opening (*stoma*). The size of the stoma may vary in size and colour. It will be quite red and swollen, but may become smaller and turn pink. A specialist bag is fitted over the stoma to collect faeces. It may still be possible for a person who has a temporary stoma to pass faeces in the normal way.

SPECIALIST ADVICE

Before and after the operation, the person will be cared for by a specialist stoma nurse. The best position for the stoma will be discussed, although it may not always be possible to decide on the site beforehand. The nurse will also provide information about the operation and advice on aftercare. For further information, contact the British Colostomy Association (*see page 176*).

AFTERCARE

A stoma should not prevent a person from leading a normal life. Stoma bags are very well designed and are not noticeable even under shorts or a swimsuit. If the correct aftercare is given, normal bowel movement should return, enabling the person to resume a full and active life. The person will need to follow specialist advice on changing the bag, skin care and diet. As the carer, you can help by making sure that there is an adequate supply of bags – these are usually prescribed.

Stoma bag

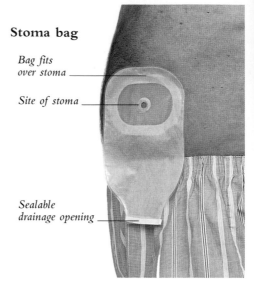

Bag fits over stoma

Site of stoma

Sealable drainage opening

Stoma bag The specialist stoma nurse will show your relative how to change the bag (*see below*). There are different designs available.

Skin care Your relative will be shown how to wash and dry around the stoma and how to identify infection.

Diet Advice will be given on identifying and cutting out foods that cause problems.

CHANGING A STOMA BAG

The bag is usually changed twice a day. Allow your relative privacy, and ensure that he has everything he requires. For the procedure he will need a bowl of warm water, soap, a towel, a replacement bag and a disposal bag, which should be provided.

The normal procedure is as follows:
♦ the stoma bag is removed and placed in the disposal bag;
♦ the stoma and surrounding area is cleaned with warm water and soap, and dried thoroughly;
♦ the new bag is attached.

CHAPTER 11

HOME FROM HOSPITAL

Your role as a carer may begin when your relative is
discharged from hospital. Before this happens, the hospital should
ensure that you have all the resources you need
to provide adequate aftercare.

AFTERCARE

Planning aftercare will be easier if you find out as
much as possible about your relative's condition and the type of
hospital treatment she has undergone. If you are caring for your
relative full-time, you may need professional assistance or part-
time help from a volunteer carer. In some situations, the special
facilities and services of a day centre may provide the
psychological and physical care your relative needs, and can also
offer you advice, support and some relief from your role.

REHABILITATION AND CONVALESCENCE

A major operation or illness may have a profound
emotional effect on your relative, especially if she has restricted
mobility and is dependent on others for the first time in
her adult life. She may also take time to adjust to being back
at home, particularly if she has been in hospital
for a long period of time.

LEAVING HOSPITAL

YOU AND YOUR RELATIVE should be consulted from the outset by the hospital about arrangements for discharge; these arrangements may even begin before your relative goes into hospital or when she is admitted. As the main carer, you will be told when to collect her from hospital, how to care for her at home, how to administer medicines and what follow-up visits are required.

ENSURING YOUR NEEDS ARE MET

The welfare of your relative and yourself is paramount in the discharge procedure. You both have rights: your relative according to the Patient's Charter (*see page 173*) and you according to the Carers Act (*see page 172*). You both have the right to complain if you are dissatisfied.

Hospital staff Firstly, speak to the nurse in charge or, if this fails, to the hospital manager.

Complaints procedure If you are still not satisfied, make a formal complaint according to the hospital's procedures.

Specialist help Seek help from the ward staff, your GP or local Community Health Council (CHC) on how to make a complaint. The Patient's Association and the Health Service Ombudsman (*see page 177*) will also be able to advise you.

BEFORE YOUR RELATIVE IS DISCHARGED

Hospital staff should only discharge a patient when they are satisfied that there is someone to care for her at home. They should always consult the patient about this, and you, as the main carer. You will need to liaise with various members of staff, such as the nurse in charge, the social worker and the doctor, in planning your relative's discharge and aftercare. You should only agree to allow her to come home when you are altogether satisfied with the arrangements.

QUESTIONS YOU SHOULD ASK THE HOSPITAL STAFF

Do not be afraid to ask questions about your relative's condition and the type of care she needs. Find out:
◆ what medicines she needs, how frequently they are required and how they should be administered;
◆ whether the medicines or the treatments have any side effects; if so, how these should be managed;
◆ how to carry out specific moving and handling manoeuvres, on your own or with help;
◆ how to cope should things go wrong.

PREPARATIONS THE HOSPITAL STAFF SHOULD MAKE

Before your relative leaves hospital, a member of staff will consult you, the main carer, and advise you when to collect her. They will also:
◆ inform the GP and district nurse of the discharge, and explain your relative's condition and likely needs;
◆ order the medicines for her immediate aftercare;
◆ arrange any specialised aftercare services, such as physiotherapy or occupational therapy;
◆ if necessary, arrange transport home;
◆ give you instructions regarding the aftercare and follow-up visits to the hospital;
◆ advise your relative when she can return to work.

PREPARING THE HOME

BEFORE YOUR RELATIVE LEAVES HOSPITAL, you need to ensure that you have the necessary resources and skills to provide adequate care. You should find out from the nurse in charge or the doctor exactly what is required of you. Once you are satisfied that you can undertake the caring role, you can make preparations for your relative's return home. (*See also* Being a Carer, *pages 13–28*).

PREPARING YOURSELF FOR CARING

Before you feel confident that you can provide adequate care, ask yourself the following questions:

◆ Do I fully understand why my relative was admitted to hospital and what treatments she received there?

◆ Am I physically and mentally capable of caring for my relative day and night?

◆ Who do I turn to in an emergency? Do I have the telephone numbers of the GP (or on-call hospital doctor) and district nursing service?

◆ Do I have enough support from other people, such as a friend, relative or volunteer carer, where necessary, to help look after my relative?

◆ What effect will the caring role have on other members of my household?

◆ Is the home sufficiently equipped? For example, are special toilet facilities, or any special aids, such as a wheelchair, needed?

If you are unsure about any of the above, you should seek the advice of the nursing staff or your relative's GP before agreeing to take on the caring role.

PRACTICAL ARRANGEMENTS AT HOME

Before your relative leaves hospital, you should make thorough preparations at home.

Preparing her room Ensure that your relative's bedroom is clean and comfortable and that it is not too hot or too cold. The layout of the room should be practical, with bedside items to hand (*see page 52*).

Preparing a meal Have a light meal ready as she may be hungry, but bear in mind dietary restrictions.

Organising visitors Stagger visits from family and friends. Talk to your relative to see if she feels up to seeing people, bearing in mind that she may feel tired.

PROLONGED ILLNESSES

Caring for someone with a prolonged illness, such as cancer or kidney disease, can be particularly difficult. Your relative will require a lot of emotional support, especially if she is undergoing intensive treatment, such as chemotherapy or dialysis. The closer you are to someone, the more difficult it can be, so it is advisable to seek outside support.

Support groups Organisations such as Macmillan Cancer Relief, Marie Curie Cancer Care or the Parkinson's Disease Society (*see pages 175–6*) offer advice and support to the affected person, and the family and friends. A support group for carers, such as Carers National Association (*see page 174*), may be able to put you and your relative in contact with others in a similar situation.

REHABILITATION

AFTER YOUR RELATIVE COMES OUT OF HOSPITAL, she may not be able to carry out some day-to-day tasks, such as having a bath or cooking for herself. You will need to assess the level of help she requires but, where possible, you should allow her to be independent. She may also have been prescribed treatment, such as physiotherapy, to take place at home, or at a day centre or hospital.

EMOTIONAL SUPPORT

Try to be sensitive to how your relative is feeling, particularly if she has experienced a major operation or an illness that required lengthy treatment. If she has had a life-changing operation or illness, she may benefit from outside support, such as counselling, to overcome any distress.

Gathering information
Find out as much as you can from the hospital staff about your relative's illness and the likely effects of the treatment she has recently undergone.

Seeking support
Various support groups have been established to help people care for specific conditions. Ask your GP or district nurse to put you in touch with one for help and advice, or telephone the relevant organisation directly for information (*see pages 174–77*).

RE-ESTABLISHING A DAILY ROUTINE

You will need to establish a routine that will ease your relative back into home life and help her to regain her health. Her daily timetable should be based on the information supplied by the hospital staff and on her individual needs. Bear in mind the following points, when working out a routine:
◆ how much rest she needs;
◆ what type of diet she requires;
◆ what she is physically capable of doing;
◆ what medication she takes;
◆ any specially devised aftercare programme, such as physiotherapy exercises (*see opposite*);
◆ follow-up treatments at the hospital and check-up visits from her GP and district nurse.

HELPING YOUR RELATIVE TO ADJUST

Once your relative is home, bear in mind her physical and emotional needs. She is likely to be too weak to carry out all the daily activities she undertook before going into hospital. She may feel insecure or even confused about being out of the routine of the hospital ward. Patience is required while she adjusts to the new location and a different way of doing things.

Rest Encourage her to take things slowly. She should rest for at least an hour in the afternoon, and catnap whenever she is tired.

Exercise If she is mobile, encourage her to take gentle exercise, even if it is only walking about indoors.

Companionship Try not to leave her alone for long periods, as she may feel isolated after being in a busy hospital ward. Although it is good for her to receive visitors, make sure she is ready for this. If possible, find time to talk to her about how she feels, and be encouraging and reassuring.

TREATMENTS AND THERAPIES

Rehabilitation means restoring an individual to normal function after a disease or injury. This process can take a long time and may require your relative to undergo regular treatments and therapies:
- as part of her treatment, your relative may be shown exercises that she can carry out herself;
- as the main carer, you may be taught simple techniques that you can regularly administer at home;
- a qualified therapist might visit your home to treat your relative;
- your relative may go for treatment at a day centre, which might also be linked to a hospital.

DAY CENTRES

Many day centres are specially equipped for elderly and disabled people and those recovering from an accident or operation. Treatment may be carried out at one of these centres if, for example, the use of specialist equipment or the skills of trained staff are required. Day centres also allow your relative to meet people who have similar needs, and give you, the carer, the chance to have a break.

THE RANGE OF THERAPIES

Following a thorough assessment of your relative's condition, the most effective treatment is prescribed.
Physiotherapy This is a combination of exercises prescribed by a physiotherapist for the patient's individual needs. The exercises are used to strengthen and heal parts of the body in conjunction with heat treatments or ultrasound, for example.
Hydrotherapy These are exercise sessions that take place in a swimming pool. Water reduces the pull of gravity on the injured part of the body, making movement easier and so reducing pain.
Occupational therapy This form of therapy helps a person to relearn everyday skills that have been lost as a result of illness or injury, such as dressing, bathing and preparing meals. It is particularly useful for stroke patients or for those who are otherwise disabled.
Speech therapy This range of exercises is designed to help someone overcome a language or speech difficulty (*see page 39*).

PHYSIOTHERAPY AT HOME

A physiotherapist will demonstrate techniques to help your relative strengthen her limbs and improve dexterity.

Hand therapy
Special items, such as putty balls, can be manipulated by hand to improve dexterity and strengthen wrist and hand movement.

Limb therapy This is effective for someone who has restricted movement. A common exercise may require you, the carer, to hold the limb (at the wrist and elbow, or ankle and knee) and move it upwards, exercising all the joints without pushing beyond the natural movement of the limb.

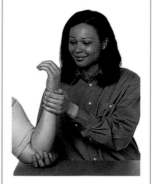

Physiotherapy exercises
You can help your relative by carrying out gentle limb therapy.

HOSPITAL DAY TREATMENTS

ADVANCES IN MEDICAL TECHNOLOGY have helped to speed up treatments, allowing a patient to be admitted to hospital as a day case. In some situations a general anaesthetic may be given, while other procedures may be carried out under a local anaesthetic or sedation. You and your relative will be told what the treatment involves, and what aftercare is required.

WHY DAY TREATMENTS ARE CARRIED OUT

Many disorders can be treated in a hospital's out-patient department. Some day procedures are also required to investigate a condition to see if an operation is needed or to give treatment following an operation. Understanding the treatment will help you to provide the best aftercare.

A GUIDE TO THE TREATMENTS AND AFTER-EFFECTS		
TREATMENT	**WHAT HAPPENS**	**AFTER-EFFECTS**
Barium X-ray	Barium is a substance that shows up on an X-ray. The patient swallows a barium "meal", which is then X-rayed (as it progresses through the intestinal tract) to investigate the bowel and rectum. Barium may also be given as an enema.	White faeces may be passed. The patient may become constipated.
MRI scan	Magnetic Resonance Imaging (MRI) uses magnetic fields and radio waves to make detailed cross-sectional pictures of the head and body, which are translated by a computer into high-quality images. The patient will be asked to remove any metal objects, and to lie as still as possible on a couch that moves through the scanner. She will hear instructions from the nurse through headphones.	The scan is painless and there are no after-effects.
Keyhole surgery	For some conditions, this is an alternative to major surgery. Tiny viewing instruments (*scopes*) are passed through small incisions in the body, then manipulated to examine and remove tissue and tumours. Typical procedures are treatment of some hernias, and removing cartilage from a knee joint.	There will be some pain and discomfort, but recuperation is swift because the surgery is relatively minimal.

A GUIDE TO THE TREATMENTS AND AFTER-EFFECTS

TREATMENT	WHAT HAPPENS	AFTER-EFFECTS
Chemotherapy	This treatment of cancer or infection may involve the injection of drugs through a vein in order to destroy abnormal cells. The first sessions usually take place in a cancer (*oncology*) unit; thereafter, they may be continued in an out-patient department and sometimes at home. In other instances, only tablets are required to be taken.	Vomiting (*see page 70*) and diarrhoea (*see page 108*) can leave the patient feeling weak and tired. Hair loss may occur.
Radiotherapy	This treats cancer through special X-rays directed at the affected part of the body to destroy the diseased or unwanted tissue. Radiotherapy may be used in combination with chemotherapy to treat some cancers.	Vomiting (*see page 70*) and diarrhoea (*see page 108*) can leave the patient feeling weak and tired.
Kidney dialysis	A procedure designed to remove harmful toxic elements from the blood and excess fluid from the body as treatment for kidney failure. Nurses or technicians operate a dialysis machine and can train the carer and relative to carry out the procedure at home.	Hunger, thirst and occasional confusion.
Gastroscopy	Long, flexible viewing instruments (*gastroscopes*) are passed through the mouth and used to investigate conditions of the stomach. A doctor views the stomach lining and makes a diagnosis.	Patients often complain of a sore throat and/or wind for a day or two after this procedure.
Cystoscopy	A method of examining the bladder: a viewing instrument (*cystoscope*) is inserted into the urethra to investigate blood in the urine and other related conditions.	Discomfort may occur for 24 hours and some blood may be passed. Drinking plenty of fluids helps prevent infection and makes it easier to pass urine.
Casts	Someone with a dislocation or broken bone may need day treatment to change a cast. Plaster of Paris or acrylic is moulded and shaped, while wet; once dry and rigid, it supports the injured part while it heals.	Check circulation in the fingers or toes. If they are cold, blue or tingle ("pins and needles"), seek medical advice.

CONVALESCENCE

RECOVERY FROM AN ILLNESS OR OPERATION may leave your relative immobile and restricted in what she is able to do. This often leads to boredom, frustration and depression. You may be able to help by encouraging pastimes that will keep her busy, and her mind active. These activities can help her focus on regaining good health and maximum independence.

ITEMS THAT AID RECOVERY

There are many aids on the market that can help your relative to overcome physical difficulties (*see page 177*).

Book stand A light, folding book stand prevents a weak person having to hold a book.

Magnifier This is a visual aid that helps someone with impaired vision to read and carry out detailed work.

Knitting machine This is designed to enable a disabled person to knit with one hand.

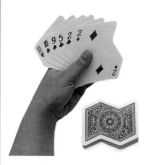

Crooked cards Useful for someone who cannot grip.

RECREATIONAL ACTIVITIES

As soon as your relative is well enough, try to introduce activities that encourage a more positive state of mind. Hobbies, games and gentle exercise will greatly improve the later stages of recovery by providing mental and physical stimulation, offering a welcome diversion from immobility, and helping to boost confidence.

HOBBIES AND INTERESTS

As your relative begins to make progress, incorporate a hobby or interest into her daily routine. If she is an elderly or disabled person, she may be able to resume a hobby with the use of appropriate aids. Equipment such as a kneeling frame, for example, allows a gardener to lower and raise herself with ease.

PLAYING GAMES

Playing cards or board games, and doing puzzles and jigsaws, are pastimes that you can enjoy together. These activities can help to keep your relative's mind alert, lift her spirits and encourage gentle motion of the upper body.

GENTLE EXERCISE

Encourage your relative to walk very short distances, then build on this according to her progress. If she is not able to walk, a short car ride will at least give her an opportunity to leave the house.

HANDICRAFTS

Crafts, such as knitting, painting and model-making, are absorbing for those who like working with their hands. These activities can be very therapeutic and are ideal for those whose mobility is restricted.

CHAPTER 12

CARE SKILLS

Part of your role may involve caring for your
relative while he has a long- or short-term illness.
As with all aspects of caring, looking after an ill person at
home requires common sense. Your main aims are to make sure
that your relative is comfortable and, where possible, to help in
alleviating any painful or distressing symptoms.
For example, if he can't get out of bed, something as simple as
keeping the room clean and well-ventilated may help to make
him feel better or if, for example, he has a condition that causes
breathing difficulties, you may be able to help by making
sure that he is in a comfortable position.

PRACTICAL SKILLS

The pages that follow give you a basic
understanding of the practical skills you need to look after
someone who is ill: how to take someone's temperature and
measure his pulse rate, how to relieve uncomfortable symptoms
and what information to record and pass on to the doctor.
There is also a guide to the type
of medication that is likely to be prescribed and how it
should be administered. If you are unable to deal with any aspect
of this type of caring, are concerned about your relative's
symptoms, or are unclear on any aspects of his medication, always
seek the advice of a healthcare professional,
such as a GP or district nurse.

TEMPERATURE CHANGES

A HEALTHY BODY MAINTAINS a constant temperature of between 36–37°C (96.8–98.6°F) by achieving a balance between the heat it produces and the heat it loses. If this balance is disturbed, a body temperature outside the normal range will result. This is often a sign of illness, so you will need to seek medical help and, in the meantime, try to alleviate any symptoms.

RECOGNISING AN ABNORMAL TEMPERATURE

If the body temperature falls below 36°C (96.8°F) or rises above 37°C (98.6°F), there may be clear signs (*see below*). Pulse and breathing rates may also indicate an abnormal temperature (*see page 128*).

SIGNS OF A VERY LOW TEMPERATURE

The person will feel cold and may be:
- shivering;
- pale;
- confused.

SIGNS OF A HIGH TEMPERATURE

The person will feel hot and may:
- have flushed cheeks;
- be sweating;
- be shivering.

WHY CHANGES OCCUR

An extreme rise or fall in temperature can occur if the body's heat regulating mechanism fails.

Low temperature A drop in temperature below 35°C (95°F) (*hypothermia*) occurs when the body loses more heat than it can produce. This can occur outdoors in very cold weather conditions, and indoors if preventive measures are not taken (*see page 129*).

High temperature This is part of the body's natural defence mechanism (*see page 56*) for fighting infection. The increase in temperature above 37°C (98.6°F) (*pyrexia*), helps to destroy many bacteria and viruses.

THERMOMETERS

Mercury and digital thermometers are the most commonly used. The former indicates temperature by means of a mercury level, the latter by a digital reading.

Mercury thermometer

Mercury level

Normal temperature range

A reading outside the 36–37°C (96.8–98.6°F) range can be a danger sign

Temperature
- 36–37°C (96.8–98.6°F) = normal
- above 37°C (98.6°F) = fever
- below 35°C (95°F) = hypothermia

Digital reading

Digital thermometer

TAKING A TEMPERATURE

Taking the temperature orally is the most common and effective method. If, for any reason, this is not possible (*see right*), the reading should be taken under the armpit (*see overleaf*). You should, however, let the GP know that you used this method as it is less accurate. You should never take the temperature via the rectum; this method should only be carried out by a doctor or nurse and is rarely necessary.

TAKING A TEMPERATURE BY MOUTH

1 Clean the thermometer by rinsing it in cold water and drying it with a clean cloth. If you are using a mercury thermometer, shake it until the mercury level is at the bottom of the scale. If you are using a digital thermometer, clean it, switch it on, then wait for the screen to go blank.

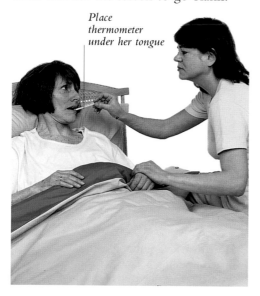

Place thermometer under her tongue

2 Place the thermometer under the person's tongue and ask her to close her lips securely to hold it in place.

WHEN NOT TO USE THE MOUTH

Taking the temperature by mouth is not safe or effective if someone:
- is unconscious;
- is confused or mentally impaired;
- is a baby, or a child aged under six;
- is suffering from a jaw injury;
- is susceptible to convulsions;
- has a cough or blocked nose;
- has recently had a hot or cold drink.

3 Leave a mercury thermometer in the person's mouth for two minutes. Leave a digital thermometer until it bleeps.

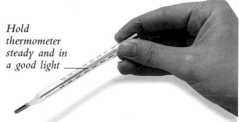

Hold thermometer steady and in a good light

4 Remove the thermometer and record the temperature by noting the mercury level or digital reading.

5 Shake the mercury back down or turn the digital thermometer off.

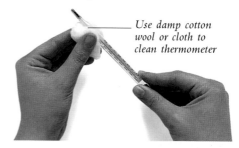

Use damp cotton wool or cloth to clean thermometer

6 Wipe the thermometer clean and return it to its case.

TAKING A TEMPERATURE UNDER THE ARMPIT

1 Rinse the thermometer in cold water and dry it with a clean cloth. Shake the mercury down to the bottom of the scale or, if you are using a digital thermometer, switch it on.

2 Make sure the thermometer and the skin under the armpit are dry. Ask the person to keep still.

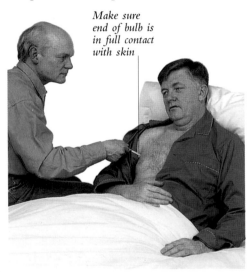

Make sure end of bulb is in full contact with skin

3 Place the thermometer in the person's armpit and ask him to fold his forearm across his chest.

4 Leave a mercury thermometer in place for two minutes. Leave a digital thermometer until it bleeps.

5 Record the temperature by noting the mercury level or digital reading.

6 Shake the mercury back down or turn the digital thermometer off. Wipe the thermometer clean and return it to its case.

BREATHING AND PULSE RATES

While taking a temperature, you should check your relative's breathing and pulse rates as an increase or decrease in these can also indicate a temperature change. The information can then be recorded and given to the GP, along with the temperature reading.

Monitor breathing At rest, a person breathes in and out (one respiration) about 16 times per minute. Anything above or below this may accompany a high or low temperature. Count your relative's breaths per minute and note your findings for the GP. To get a more accurate measure, do not tell him that you are monitoring his breathing.

Check the pulse The pulse is the "wave" that courses through the body each time the heart pumps blood into the circulatory system. The normal pulse rate for a person at rest is between 60–80 beats per minute; anything above or below this level, and any change in the strength of the pulse, may accompany a high or low temperature.

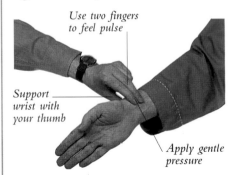

Use two fingers to feel pulse

Support wrist with your thumb

Apply gentle pressure

How to take a pulse Place your fingertips in the hollow just above the wrist creases at the base of the thumb. Count the beats for one minute and record the figure. Try to judge the strength of the pulse as well as the rhythm.

Dealing with a High Temperature

A high temperature is usually the result of an infection (*see page 54*), and may, therefore, be impossible to prevent and difficult to control.

Treating a high temperature
Your aims are to try to lower the temperature and make your relative comfortable. Call the GP if a high temperature persists or you are worried.
Offer the chance to freshen up Ask your relative if he would like a wash, and a change of clothes and bed linen.
Monitor room temperature Ensure that the room is adequately ventilated. You can use a fan, but do not overchill.
Provide fluids and food Give him plenty of cold drinks, and offer frequent mouthwashes. Loss of fluid may cause appetite loss and sluggish bowel movements, so provide light meals only.

Offer medication Paracetamol may lower the temperature – make sure that you give the correct dosage and check with the pharmacist that it does not conflict with other medication.
Cool with water Sponge your relative all over with tepid water, but do not let him get too cold. Gently dry him afterwards. Alternatively, apply a cool compress to his forehead.

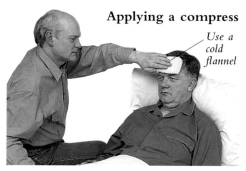

Applying a compress

Use a cold flannel

Dealing with a Low Temperature

Hypothermia can occur when the body temperature drops below 35°C (95°F) and if the surrounding temperature is especially cold. Those most at risk are elderly, immobile and ill people.

Treating hypothermia
Hypothermia is a life-threatening condition, so urgent medical help should always be sought. An elderly person should be rewarmed gradually (*see page 157*). A young, fit person can be rewarmed by having a bath.

Preventing hypothermia
Take steps to prevent your relative from getting hypothermia.
Regulate room temperature The temperature drops at night, so ensure that

the bedroom is kept at around 18°C (64.4°F). Seek advice on financial allowances for heating bills for someone with a limited income.
Provide sufficient food and drink Hot food and drink, and regular meals, are essential. If your relative is immobile, keep a flask of hot drink close by him.
Provide effective clothing Several layers of light clothing are more effective than one thick layer. Gloves and socks help to keep extremities such as fingers and toes warm. A hat prevents heat-loss from the head, especially if someone is bald or has thinning hair.
Encourage movement Exercise helps the circulation of blood. A few minutes walking around the room will help if your relative is able to do so.

BREATHING DIFFICULTIES

I F THE PERSON YOU ARE CARING FOR experiences difficulty breathing, you
should seek medical advice immediately. Breathlessness may be a symptom
of a short-term illness, such as the flu, but it could also result from a lung
condition, such as asthma, or even a heart problem. Treatments range from
self-help remedies to the use of specialist equipment.

ALLEVIATING BREATHING DIFFICULTIES

Breathing difficulties can be prevented
or minimised by considering
environmental factors, and by the
person assuming the most comfortable
and effective posture to ease breathing.

ENVIRONMENT
A room's atmosphere may aggravate
your relative's breathing difficulties. Try
to establish whether there are any
specific factors that appear to improve
or worsen the condition and, if possible,
make changes to alleviate the problem.
Ventilate rooms Hot rooms, especially
those that are centrally heated, can
aggravate respiratory problems. You can
help by making sure that:
◆ rooms are adequately ventilated;
◆ the heating is not too high;
◆ the atmosphere is not too dry
(a bowl of water placed in the room
can increase humidity).
Pinpoint allergies There may be
contributing factors to your relative's
condition. You can help by:
◆ keeping known allergens, such as
animal fur or feather pillows, away;
◆ keeping the environment as clean and
dust-free as possible.
Encourage outdoor activities Being
outdoors may help to alleviate the
problem. Encourage your relative to:
◆ go for walks in pollution-free areas;
◆ sit in the garden, if the weather allows.

POSTURE
There are various positions that a
person can assume whether in bed or
in a chair that can make breathing easier.
Your relative will probably know which
position is most comfortable, so always
listen to him. The positions include:
◆ sitting in an upright chair, supported
by pillows or a backrest;
◆ sitting upright in a bed with pillows or
a specially designed backrest (*see page 87*);
◆ leaning forwards with arms supported
on a chair or a stool, for temporary relief.

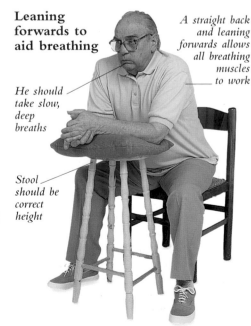

**Leaning
forwards to
aid breathing**

*A straight back
and leaning
forwards allows
all breathing
muscles
to work*

*He should
take slow,
deep
breaths*

*Stool
should be
correct
height*

MEDICATION FOR BREATHING DIFFICULTIES

Medication can vary from antibiotics for chest infections, to inhalers and oxygen for more long-term breathing difficulties.

PRESCRIBED INHALERS

Someone with a breathing difficulty, such as asthma, will be prescribed an inhaler and shown how to use it; the device enables medication to be inhaled directly into the lungs. Make sure an inhaler and a refill are always readily available. There are different types.

Preventer inhaler This is usually brown or white. A sufferer uses it regularly to prevent an attack.

Reliever inhaler This type of inhaler is usually blue. It is used during an attack to open the airways.

Spacer This device has a mouthpiece at one end and a hole for the inhaler at the other end. The inhaler is inserted into the spacer and the medication is squirted into it before being breathed in through the mouthpiece. These are often used to enable a child, elderly person or someone who is weak to inhale the medication more effectively.

Nebuliser This is a small machine that provides a larger dose of medication than an inhaler. It is only used when breathing difficulties are severe.

Using an inhaler

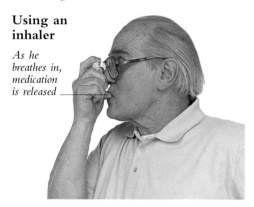

As he breathes in, medication is released

PHYSIOTHERAPY

Breathlessness may be treated with physiotherapy. Chest physiotherapy, postural drainage and breathing techniques are simple treatments that can be carried out at home. In an illness such as cystic fibrosis, these can help to minimise infection by enabling the lungs to keep clear of the sticky mucus brought on by the condition. After surgery, especially when the chest cavity has been opened, breathing exercises can help the person to regain normal breathing patterns. Whatever the condition, a physiotherapist will train you in the techniques that are suitable for your relative's age and illness. Treatment may be daily, or more often for serious conditions.

STEAM INHALATION

A simple home remedy for loosening phlegm and easing coughing is to add an inhalant to steaming hot water. The person then inhales the steam. Inhalation can be an effective treatment for colds, flu and mild bronchitis. Ask your pharmacist to recommend an inhalant.

Method Add the inhalant to a bowl of hot water, following the instructions on the bottle. Ask the person to sit down and place his face directly over the bowl. Make sure that:

◆ the water is not *boiling* hot;

◆ his face is not too close to the water. Place a towel over his head, large enough to cover his head and the bowl. Advise him to inhale for up to ten minutes, and stay with him throughout.

GIVING OXYGEN

Oxygen may be prescribed for chronic chest or heart complaints.

For intermittent use Oxygen is supplied by a cylinder in the home and given via a mask.

For continuous use A machine will be installed in the home. This machine provides a continuous supply of oxygen to the person through nasal tubes.

To aid mobility In addition to a large cylinder, the person may be given a portable cylinder, enabling her to walk around, climb stairs and leave the house and still receive oxygen.

Oxygen cylinder

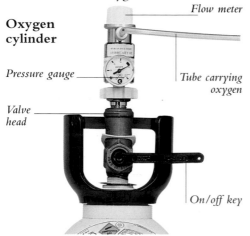

Flow meter

Pressure gauge

Valve head

Tube carrying oxygen

On/off key

OXYGEN PRECAUTIONS

Always follow instructions carefully:
◆ only give oxygen at the rate prescribed;
◆ monitor oxygen level;
◆ check level of water in any humidifier;
◆ keep cylinders away from fires, naked flames, electrical toys, grease and oil;
◆ do not smoke near oxygen cylinders;
◆ always keep spare supplies;
◆ store cylinders in a cool place.

GIVING OXYGEN BY MASK

1 Before giving oxygen, read the pressure gauge to check how much oxygen the cylinder contains.

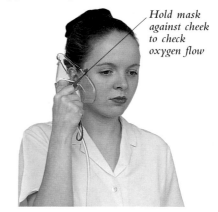

Hold mask against cheek to check oxygen flow

2 Connect the tube of the mask to the cylinder, as instructed. Use the key to open the cylinder valve and adjust the rate of flow of oxygen according to the instructions. Check that the oxygen is flowing by holding the mask near to your cheek.

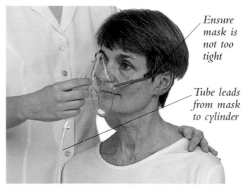

Ensure mask is not too tight

Tube leads from mask to cylinder

3 Arrange the mask over the person's nose and mouth. Record the amount of oxygen given in litres per minute. You may be provided with a mask that delivers a fixed percentage of oxygen.

MEDICATION

THERE ARE TWO CATEGORIES of medication: those that require a doctor's prescription and those that do not. You should have an understanding of why your relative needs to take any medication, and be aware of potential side effects. Your main aims are to make sure medication is taken correctly and, wherever possible, allow your relative to take it by himself.

MEDICATION GUIDELINES

When assisting with medication, follow the basic rules:
- check you have the correct medication;
- only give medication to the person for whom it has been prescribed;
- make sure the exact quantity prescribed is taken at the recommended times.

PRESCRIBED MEDICATION

Follow the GP's instructions and always read the label and accompanying leaflets. Contact the GP's surgery or the pharmacist for advice if necessary.

OVER-THE-COUNTER MEDICATION

There has been a huge increase in the availability of over-the-counter drugs that do not require a prescription. These are available at supermarkets and local shops, as well as at chemists. If your relative is already on medication, or you have any doubts about the drugs you are buying, you should always seek the advice of a pharmacist or GP.

SIDE EFFECTS OF MEDICATION

Read the leaflet supplied with the medication or check with the GP and the pharmacist about any side effects.

Drowsiness The person will be advised not to drink alcohol, drive or operate machinery.

Diet The GP or the pharmacist should advise if any dietary restrictions need to be observed.

Adverse reactions Side effects, such as diarrhoea, vomiting, dizziness, skin rashes and any other unexpected problems should be reported to the GP.

DO'S & DON'TS

✅ **Do** wash your hands (*see page 56*) before and after giving medication.

✅ **Do** check the expiry date if the medication has not been used for some time.

✅ **Do** store medication in a child-proof container, especially when it is stored in the fridge.

✅ **Do** follow storage instructions.

✅ **Do** dispose of needles and syringes correctly (*see page 58*).

✅ **Do** return unwanted prescription medication to a GP or pharmacist.

❌ **Don't** give the medication if it has changed colour or has turned cloudy.

❌ **Don't** give the medication if you are unable to read the label.

❌ **Don't** store different pills in one bottle.

❌ **Don't** decant from one bottle into another.

TYPES OF MEDICATION

Liquids Always shake the bottle to mix the constituents thoroughly. Follow the instructions on the bottle and use the correct size of measuring spoon. Don't use the medicine if it has changed colour or turned cloudy.

Tablets These can be crushed and mixed with honey or jam, unless there are dietary restrictions. Sugar-coated tablets and those that have a shiny shell should be swallowed whole, if possible, with a drink.

Capsules These should not be broken open as they are designed to dissolve slowly in the stomach. They are easier to swallow if placed at the back of the tongue and taken with a drink.

Powders These can be stirred and dissolved in liquids such as water or milk. Mixing them with foods, such as jam or honey, can also make them more palatable, but check that no dietary restrictions apply.

Suppositories and pessaries Suppositories are inserted into the rectum; pessaries into the vagina. The person should insert these according to medical instruction. Do not administer them yourself unless properly instructed.

Creams/lotions Some lotions and creams contain powerful drugs, such as steroids. Always follow the instructions on the tube or bottle. It is advisable to wear latex gloves (*see page 57*) when applying some creams and lotions.

Inhalers These enable a person to inhale drugs to alleviate breathing difficulties (*see page 131*). Colour coding enables you to differentiate between the different types.

Needles A person who needs regular medication by injection is usually taught how to do this himself. Ensure that the dosage is correct and that needles are disposed of safely (*see page 58*).

MONITORING DOSAGE

The person you are caring for may be on more than one type of medication, and knowing when to take each one can be confusing. To help, a pharmacist can supply the medication in a way that makes it easy to monitor dosage. Normally, he will divide a week's supply into separate daily doses, either in compartmentalised cassettes or blister packs, so that the person can see at a glance which medication to take and when to take it. Each compartment or pack is labelled with the day and the time the named dose is to be taken.

Advantages This system enables you to:
◆ monitor dosages of medication, while allowing your relative to be independent;
◆ minimise the risk of conflicting medications being taken together;
◆ in an emergency, provide instant information about which medication the person has taken.

ADMINISTERING EYE, NOSE AND EAR DROPS

Medications for the eye, nose and ear usually come in the form of drops. These are sterile and should always be used before the expiry date on the package. If only one eye or ear is affected, make sure that you apply drops to the correct side, as it can be dangerous to use medication on healthy organs. When applying eye drops, do not allow the dropper to come into contact with the eye as this can often cause infection to spread. Wash the dropper should it become contaminated. It is common for steroids or drugs such as antibiotics and antihistamines to be given in eye, nose or ear drop form.

APPLYING EYE DROPS

1 Stand behind the person. Ask him to lean his head back against you and look up.

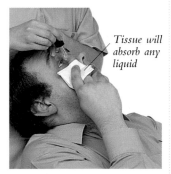

Tissue will absorb any liquid

2 Give him a tissue to hold against his cheek. Gently pull back the upper eyelid. Squeeze the correct dosage into the space between the lower eyelid and the eyeball, near to the inside corner of the eye.

3 The person will automatically close his eye. Ask him to blink a couple of times. This disperses the eye drop over the whole surface of the eye.

APPLYING NASAL DROPS

1 Ask the person to blow his nose so that any blockage is cleared before applying the drops.

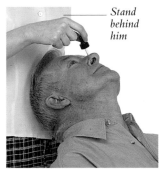

Stand behind him

2 Ask him to tilt his head as far back as possible. Insert the tip of the dropper just inside the nostril and squeeze out the correct dosage. Repeat this procedure for the other nostril.

3 Ask him to sniff to disperse the drops within the nasal cavity. Advise him to stay in the same position for a short while and to refrain from blowing his nose for at least 20 minutes.

APPLYING EAR DROPS

1 Ask the person to tilt her head so that the affected ear is uppermost.

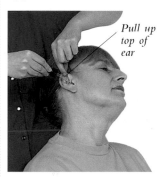

Pull up top of ear

2 Grip top of the ear. Hold the dropper just above the opening. Allow the drops to trickle into the ear canal.

3 Ask the person to keep her head still, in the same position, for a few minutes.

4 Place a piece of cotton wool just over the opening to the ear. Under no circumstances should the cotton wool be pushed into the ear canal.

WOUND CARE

A WOUND IS A BREAK IN THE SKIN, and may be the result of an injury, disease or an operation. The kind of care needed depends on the size and severity of the wound. If the wound is large and gaping, you should seek professional help. Wounds due to an operation, or conditions such as varicose ulcers, may require regular aftercare, and this will usually be carried out by a district nurse.

THE HEALING PROCESS

When any part of the body has been damaged, as a result of, for example, a cut, wound or pressure sore, tissues adjacent to the injured area will begin to repair the damage. If tissue has been lost, as occurs with a burn or an abscess, for example, or if the affected area has been contaminated in any way, it will take longer for the body to heal itself.

The body repairs the damaged area in the following way:
◆ the wound bleeds and the ruptured area is filled with blood that clots quickly, then dries to form a scab;

◆ white blood cells begin to destroy and remove dead and damaged tissue;

◆ cells grow rapidly in the clotted blood;

◆ firm, fibrous tissues form across the wound and may become a scar.

TREATING A WOUND

As a carer, you may be asked to help the district nurse to dress a wound or have to deal with a wound in an emergency. It is a good idea to keep sterile dressings (*see page 162*) in your basic first-aid kit at home. Your main aims when dressing a wound are:
◆ to prevent bacteria entering the wound;
◆ to hasten healing and alleviate pain.

PREVENTING INFECTION

To prevent the wound becoming infected, always:
◆ wash your hands before treatment (*see page 56*);
◆ wear sterile latex gloves, if possible (*see page 57*);
◆ clean the area so that dirt is washed away;
◆ cover the wound with a dressing, preferably sterile;
◆ dry the surrounding skin with a clean towel;
◆ secure dressings properly and keep them dry;
◆ dispose of used dressings and gloves (*see page 58*).
An infected wound Seek medical advice if the wound begins to ooze, the skin around the wound becomes red, there is swelling or discomfort, or the person complains of feeling hot or being in pain.

AIDING THE HEALING PROCESS

Babies and children heal much more rapidly than someone who is unwell or elderly. Those with an underlying condition that requires drugs such as steroids, or others that suppress their immunity, may heal less quickly.

What the body requires In order for a wound to heal, a person needs to be physically healthy. If a wound fails to heal, it may be because of an underlying condition, such as anaemia, and the advice of a healthcare professional, such as a GP or district nurse, should be sought.

CHAPTER 13

PALLIATIVE CARE

The aim of palliative care is to ensure that a person
who has a seemingly incurable condition suffers as little as
possible, and that all her physical, psychological and spiritual needs
are satisfied. The onus is on relieving and easing each symptom of
the illness, rather than curing the disease itself, and on
facilitating a peaceful and dignified death.
Palliative care is not necessarily short-term – where
the illness is degenerative, care may stretch over many years.
Many people prefer to die at home in familiar surroundings and
in the company of their families; this is usually only feasible
if specialist help is provided by a GP or district nurse, with
adequate support from, for example, a hospice, and other
appropriate healthcare professionals.

CLOSE RELATIONSHIPS

Although caring for someone who is dying is
stressful and upsetting, it can give people the chance to
say goodbye properly. It may also reunite a family, forge friendships
and provide an opportunity to express affection. Close
relationships between the carer, the family and friends
are likely to continue after the death, and can be
a great source of comfort and support
to those who are grieving.

FACING DEATH

FINDING OUT THAT SOMEONE is going to die brings with it a wide range of emotions. Your dying relative may fear death, pain or simply the unknown. You may have fears about seeing someone who is close to you suffer, and you may worry about being left alone once she has died. These fears are understandable; talking about them openly may help you begin to cope.

DO'S & DON'TS

The quality of care you provide will improve if you also look after your own needs.

✓ **Do** acknowledge your own grief. It is a sign of human strength, not human failing.

✓ **Do** turn to healthcare professionals for their support, and take advantage of their experience and expertise.

✓ **Do** seek the help of volunteer carers.

✗ **Don't** feel guilty if you are angry or frightened that your relative is dying. These emotions are natural, but try confiding in others rather than depressing your relative.

✗ **Don't** bottle up your emotions as this may create even more stress.

✗ **Don't** regard yourself as useless. You are providing essential support in a difficult time of need.

WHEN THE NEWS IS BROKEN

You may be one of the first people to be informed that your relative is terminally ill, but it is the responsibility of the healthcare professional, not you, to inform her of this. You will, however, need to be prepared for how you handle this delicate subject.

Be informed If possible, try to be present when your relative receives the news: by listening and learning about her condition you may be able to provide comfort and support later.

Be honest If your relative asks you to expand on any detail, try to tell the truth as sensitively as possible. If there are any questions you cannot answer, seek the advice of a healthcare professional.

Be discreet Your relative may not wish to discuss death, or may even refuse to believe she is dying. If you need to talk about it, discuss the issue with the rest of the family or with an outsider, such as the GP.

THE IMPORTANCE OF COMMUNICATION

As death approaches, it is important that the dying person is encouraged to share her feelings.

Talking Do not be put off if she is unable to speak; listening to you talking can be very soothing.

Listening If she is able to express her wishes and sentiments, listen patiently and carefully; this is one of the most important things you can do for her.

Writing If she finds it difficult to talk, suggest that she writes down her feelings.

Touching Hold her hand; this can soothe anxieties and communicate reassurance and affection.

Counselling Your relative may benefit from talking to someone outside her family and close friends, such as a professional counsellor (*see page 22*).

STAGES OF GRIEF

AFTER THE INITIAL SHOCK of learning that someone is terminally ill, there are various emotions and stages of grief that may affect those concerned. It can be an unsettling time; one moment you may be deeply emotional, the next you may feel numb. You will be able to cope better, and support your relative more effectively, if you are as open as possible about your feelings.

DEALING WITH GRIEF		
EMOTION	HOW IT IS EXPRESSED	HOW TO DEAL WITH IT
Denial	◆ Your dying relative may reject the diagnosis, even after many doctors have been consulted. Be prepared to acknowledge that she may never accept the reality. ◆ It is often easier to ignore the implications of death than to face up to the reality of it. Some people may conceal shock and try to cope by behaving as if nothing has happened.	◆ You should listen patiently and sensitively to your relative. If she does not acknowledge that she is dying, do not press the point; she will deal with it in her own way. ◆ Discuss your feelings, if possible, with your dying relative and close family and friends. If everyone is able to accept the reality, this could reduce the emotional stress that is felt later.
Anger	◆ The dying person is likely to feel angry because she is afraid of death. She may direct her anger at you and others who care for her, which may be difficult to handle. She may also become irritable and depressed. ◆ You and others who are close to your relative may feel angry that she is dying.	◆ Accept that anger is a natural step towards your relative accepting her death, and try not to take personally any anger that is directed at you. ◆ Anger can be a good way for both of you to vent your feelings. Ask healthcare professionals for advice on how best to deal with angry confrontations.
Acceptance	◆ Having worked through denial and anger, your relative may finally accept that she is dying. ◆ She may ask for your help with practical arrangements, such as making a will. ◆ She may feel ready to have visitors and make the most of the time she has left.	◆ Offer to help your relative to put her affairs in order. Reassure her that you will try to simplify issues and take responsibility for what has to be done. ◆ Encourage visitors to come at a time when your relative is feeling at her best, so that she does not become agitated or exhausted.

PRACTICAL CARE

WHEN YOU ARE CARING for a dying relative, one of your main aims will be to give her the best quality of life possible. This means making sure that she is comfortable, free of pain and, to alleviate boredom and depression, has enough to keep her occupied. Always try to respect your relative's wishes and encourage her to be as independent as possible.

PROFESSIONAL SUPPORT

You may feel unable to give enough time to your relative, offer adequate care or cope with the many demands on your own. In this situation, you may need to seek part- or full-time professional help. Consult the GP for advice and information on what help is available.

Think ahead Anticipate when you might need the extra help and try to make the necessary arrangements before you find yourself in a crisis situation.

Seek short-term help Some local health authorities and charities have agencies that provide short-term care.

Seek full-time help Hospices, nursing homes or specialist organisations (*see pages 174–77*) provide care for the terminally ill, and help and advise those looking after the person.

COMFORTABLE SURROUNDINGS

If your relative is confined to bed or to the house, personal space will be extremely important to her. You can help by trying to make her feel comfortable and in control of her surroundings.

THE ROOM
For your relative's comfort, make sure her surroundings are kept clean and pleasant.
Ventilate the room A stuffy room can be unpleasant: open the windows, but avoid creating a draught.
Find the right level of light Arrange the curtains so that as much or as little light comes into the room to suit your relative's needs.
Make the room look pleasant Fresh flowers will add colour and fragrance, and liven up the room. Potpourri and scented candles may freshen the air.

VISITORS
Before encouraging friends or relatives to visit, make sure your relative wants to see them. Ideally, visits should be restricted to people with whom your relative feels comfortable. Do not be afraid to cancel visits if you feel that she is unable to cope. Remember, also, that too many visitors may put a strain on you, as the carer.
Monitor the length of visits Short, frequent visits are better than irregular, drawn-out ones that may be exhausting for your relative.
Restrict numbers of visitors One or two visitors at a time may be less overwhelming than large groups.
Prepare visitors Try to prepare visitors for your relative's appearance and attitude. They may find it awkward or feel shocked or upset if she is physically different or very depressed.

Daily Care

Encourage your relative to eat and drink, keep clean and generally look after herself. Accept, however, that she may not want to do so. Inform the GP if your relative has any uncomfortable symptoms, such as bowel problems, vomiting or pressure sores.

Eating and drinking

Eating meals She may prefer small, appetising snacks at frequent intervals rather than three large meals a day. Make a note of any changes in appetite, and report them to the healthcare professional.

Drinking fluids Even if your relative does not wish to eat, encourage her to drink plenty of fluids.

Indulgences Allow your relative to have alcohol, cigarettes or chocolate, should she request them.

Personal hygiene and appearance

Washing Encourage your relative to wash and bathe for her personal comfort and dignity. If she is confined to bed, you may be shown how to give her a bed bath (*see page 99*).

Personal grooming You can help by offering to wash and brush your relative's hair and cut her fingernails and toenails. A man may feel better if he has had a shave, and a woman may require assistance with applying make-up (*see page 101*), especially when visitors are expected.

Getting dressed Unless your relative is confined to bed, it is not necessary for her to stay in nightwear. Encourage her to get dressed, as this can give her dignity and bolster confidence.

Using the toilet Encourage your relative to get out of bed to use the toilet. If she cannot, obtain toilet aids that allow maximum independence (*see page 114*).

Living life to the full

Mobility If your relative is able, she should be encouraged to be mobile, even if this only means getting out of bed to sit in a chair.

Hobbies If she is physically able, try to stimulate interest in pastimes that you know she enjoys. This may give her pleasure, and encouragement to live the remainder of her life to the full.

Helping to Minimise Pain

A dying person's greatest fear may be the prospect of coping with pain.

Reassure your relative You can reassure your relative that from the time of diagnosis, and throughout her care, she will be given medicines to minimise pain.

Act promptly Should she suffer pain at any time, inform a healthcare professional so that the situation can be rectified as soon as possible.

Find out about specialist equipment The use of specialist equipment will be explained to you, and administered under the supervision of a healthcare professional. For example, a pain-relieving device such as a TENS (Transcutaneous Electrical Nerve Stimulator) may be recommended, or syringe pumps may be used to administer pain-relieving drugs. Speak to the GP about what is suitable.

Consider alternative therapies Your relative may prefer to try techniques such as reflexology, aromatherapy and visualisation.

TOWARDS THE END OF LIFE

As THE HEALTH OF YOUR RELATIVE DETERIORATES, you may notice signs that indicate she is dying. As life recedes, she will become weaker, sleep more frequently and for longer periods. In some cases, death may occur without warning. Your main – though perhaps daunting – aim is to make your relative's last days as peaceful and as pain-free as possible.

PLANNING AHEAD

If your relative has expressed any wishes before she dies, these should be honoured.

Living will A living will (*Advance Directive*) allows a person to refuse or express a choice on future treatment should she become too ill to do so later. Medical staff are usually sympathetic to living wills, and may offer the person counselling about the choices that are available. To avoid complications at a later stage, ensure that your relative's wishes are clear, unambiguous and witnessed. Inform family members of her wishes in case they try to intervene at a later stage. Legally, relatives have little power to change any decision that has been made.

Donor card If your relative carries a donor card, find out what her exact intentions are concerning donation.

MAKING SOMEONE COMFORTABLE

Dying is often a slow, peaceful process. Your relative may slip in and out of consciousness, or perhaps lose consciousness altogether.

Talk and hold hands Even if your relative is unconscious, she may still be able to hear and feel. Do not be afraid to talk to her or hold her hand, as this can provide comfort.

Maintain privacy Be guided by your relative's wishes and general condition.

Arrange spiritual support A visit from a spiritual adviser, such as a priest, could help give your relative the strength and courage to face death.

MAKING ARRANGEMENTS IN ADVANCE

One of the most delicate areas you may have to discuss with your relative is her funeral, but do not force the issue. If she wants to talk about it, ask if she has any preferences regarding the following:

- whether she wishes to be buried or cremated;
- the type of service: any hymns, music or readings;
- the type of headstone or memorial, and inscription;
- where the ashes should be scattered.

FIND OUT IMPORTANT INFORMATION

Find out the names, addresses and telephone numbers of people who should be notified of death and locate the following documents:

- the will;
- medical card;
- National Insurance card;
- birth and marriage certificates;
- insurance, pension and other policies;
- bank details.

ROLE OF THE VOLUNTEER CARER

THE DEMANDS ON YOU as a volunteer carer outside the family circle will be great at this time. Family members and friends of the person who is dying may need you as much as, if not more than, the person in your care, and this can be particularly stressful. To help you cope with the demands and strains of your role, bear in mind what people will expect of you during this time.

COMPLEMENTARY CARE

Your responsibility as a carer outside the family circle is to complement, not dominate, the care regime. Try to achieve a balance between supporting the needs of the dying person and those who are close to her. Allow family and friends to be involved in her care.

ESSENTIAL QUALITIES OF THE CARER

As a volunteer carer, you will need to be a source of strength and support at all times; not only to the person in your care, but also to the dying person's close family and friends.

Sensitivity and tact You will need these skills as you support the home carer, the person who is dying and her relatives. Try not to intrude into their grief, and allow the home carer to do as much or as little of the caring as she wishes. Your role is to offer only the practical and psychological help that might be required of you. Allow friends and family as much privacy as you can. Respect their wishes at all times, particularly those who are religiously or spiritually motivated.

Sympathy and patience Be as sympathetic and patient as you can. Listen to the dying person's friends and relatives if they want to talk about their feelings; leave well alone if they do not. Try to be patient when people repeat themselves, and show them that you are aware of their needs. If a person refuses to acknowledge what is happening, you should respect this.

Calmness and composure It is natural for grieving relatives to feel increasingly emotional and concerned as the dying person becomes weaker. You will need to remain calm at all times, particularly in the immediate period after the person has died, in order to provide comfort, reassurance and support.

SPIRITUAL AND CULTURAL NEEDS

You may be well aware of the dying person's spiritual views, but, if not, you may find it useful to acquaint yourself with her beliefs and customs.

Obtain information
Ask the person, or her family and close friends, about her beliefs. Obtain additional information if needed (*see page 37*).

Find out about religious customs
Consult the spiritual adviser, if there is one, so that you are aware of any particular customs.

Show respect Once you are familiar with the person's spiritual needs, try to bear them in mind at all times.

Arrange special visits
To gain the courage to face death, the person may ask you to arrange a visit from a member of his religious community, such as a priest.

WHEN DEATH OCCURS

YOU CAN NEVER REALLY PREPARE yourself fully for the moment of your relative's death. The experience will be different for everyone, and everyone will have different ways of reacting to it. Being present when someone dies is an ultimately personal, intimate and even positive experience, intrinsically bound up with your relationship with that person.

CASE STUDY

NAME: JANINE
AGE: 40

Janine had cared for her mother, Valerie, a sufferer of Alzheimer's disease, for more than five years. She had even moved into Valerie's house when she could no longer look after herself. Although Janine had often thought about her mother's death, she was not prepared for it happening suddenly.

One day, Janine found Valerie slumped on the sofa. She checked for signs of life and called her mother's GP, who later confirmed that Valerie had suffered a cardiac arrest minutes before Janine had entered the room.

As she came to terms with her mother's death, Janine realised how shocked she had been by the suddenness of it, but thinking back, she was glad that they had had so much time together before she died.

IF SOMEONE DIES AT HOME

Although death may sometimes be sudden and unexpected, it is in many instances a gentle slipping away rather than a dramatic event. Try to prepare yourself as much as possible and know what to do should your relative die at home.

HOW DO I KNOW IF SOMEONE HAS DIED?

If you are not sure whether your relative has actually passed away, the following simple checks may be useful indicators:
♦ check the pulse (*see page 128*) and look, listen and feel carefully for any signs of breathing;
♦ check the eyes, looking for signs of movement. Recheck these signs after a few minutes.

WHAT DO I DO WHEN SOMEONE HAS DIED?

Before you do anything, make sure you observe any religious customs. Inform the GP and the family and, if you feel comfortable dealing with the body and any equipment, follow the procedures below.

Call the GP When he arrives, tell him the approximate time and nature of the death so that he can produce a death certificate (*see opposite*).

Inform the family Close members of the family may wish to spend some time alone with the person before the undertaker removes the body.

Lay the body flat Remove the pillows from the bed, straighten the body and lay it flat.

Switch off equipment If there is any electrical equipment in place, turn it off. You do not need to detach any equipment from the body.

Call the undertaker The undertaker will remove any syringes or catheters and take the body to the mortuary, where it will remain until the funeral.

FINAL ARRANGEMENTS

AFTER THE DEATH, everyone involved will experience a range of emotions as they begin to come to terms with what has happened. Accept any offers of help to make funeral and other arrangements. You may feel detached as you organise the funeral and deal with formalities; it is very normal to feel this way and for the reality of the death not to sink in until later.

ARRANGEMENTS AFTER DEATH

There are various documents you will need to obtain following the person's death:
* a signed death certificate from the GP;
* the relevant details and documents for registering the death (*see right*).

With these documents you can get a death certificate from your local registry office for which there is a fee. You will need at least three copies of the death certificate for legal, insurance and banking purposes. Contact the Benefits Agency (*see page 177*) and other relevant persons to cancel any allowances.

ARRANGING THE FUNERAL

If you discussed the funeral with your relative before she died, you may already know what kind of service is required. The funeral director will:
* contact the place of burial or cremation;
* discuss the type of service you require;
* arrange a suitable date and time for the service.

You will need to:
* notify friends and relatives of the date and venue;
* organise flowers, if required, for the service;
* organise a venue for a post-funeral gathering.

TALKING TO OTHER MOURNERS

For some, the loss of a loved one may become real for the first time at the funeral.

Acknowledge the loss Talking about your relative and sharing memories with others who knew her will help the grieving process.

Celebrate life The funeral need not be a sad and solemn affair. With the help of those people who mattered most to your relative you can make it a time to celebrate the importance of her life.

REGISTERING A DEATH

You must register the death within five days. An appointment with the registrar is not necessary, but you will have to visit the office in person. The address will be in the telephone directory. You will need to provide the registrar with the following information and documentation:
* certificate of the cause of death (from the GP);
* full name (and maiden name, if relevant) and address of deceased;
* birth certificate of the deceased;
* deceased's last full-time occupation, even if she was retired;
* the name and occupation of spouse, if relevant;
* marital status of the deceased and date of birth of surviving spouse;
* medical card number, pension and benefit details of the deceased.

AFTER DEATH

THE WEEKS THAT FOLLOW the death may prove to be difficult for you as you adjust from being a full-time carer. With less to occupy you, it is easy to dwell on your loss rather than look forward to the future. Now is the time for you to enjoy the company of people who care about you and those who miss your relative, and give and receive sympathy and support.

CASE STUDY

NAME: ELIZABETH
AGE: 56

Elizabeth had been her husband's carer for two years, and she was devastated when he died. For several weeks, she felt uneasy about leaving the house, even just to go shopping, but she knew she had to start getting on with her life.

Then, one day, she saw an advertisement for an evening course in pottery. Taking her courage in her hands, Elizabeth enrolled on the course. On the first evening, she discovered she had no real talent for pottery, but she did meet Daphne, also recently widowed. The two women soon developed a firm friendship fuelled by many shared interests.

Of course Elizabeth still missed her husband and thought of him often, yet by making a determined effort she was able to maintain a fulfilling life.

GRIEVING

While you may have anticipated the grief you would feel after losing a loved one, you may have grown accustomed to suppressing your feelings in the interests of caring for the person. Although it may be difficult, the ability to express your grief is an essential part of the recovery procedure. There are many ways you can help yourself through the grieving process.

Be patient Allow yourself the time to grieve.

Be open Try not to suppress your emotions. It is far healthier to shed tears and express your grief to others.

Be honest Do not feel guilty about being relieved or angry that your relative has died; these reactions often follow the loss of someone close, particularly if the person suffered, or you cared for her for a long time.

Be positive Try not to dwell solely on feelings of loss; try to use your grief positively by expressing the joy of having known your relative.

Be resourceful There are many organisations that provide advice and counselling (*see pages 174–77*); most hospices provide bereavement counselling.

GIVING AND RECEIVING SUPPORT

Grieving is a long process and it is important that support is maintained throughout this period. Sharing and exchanging sympathy can be a great comfort and will help all concerned to grieve.

Express yourself Try to express how you feel and how you intend to cope without the person.

Reminisce Be open: others may wish to talk to you about your relative and reminisce about the past.

Be sociable Make the effort to see people. If possible, try to maintain contact with those who have helped you; their continuing support may help you adjust to your new circumstances.

CHAPTER 14

EMERGENCY CARE

As a carer you need to know what emergency
action to take if your relative is seriously ill or injured.
The following section is not a substitute for first-aid training, but
if you familiarise yourself with the techniques shown, it will help
you to administer fast and effective treatments for potentially life-
threatening conditions. Remember, you can only do what you
believe to be correct: some conditions inevitably lead to death,
even in the best medical hands. This book's companion volume,
the *First Aid Manual*, outlines all first-aid procedures; if you would
like information on courses, contact your local branch of St. John,
St. Andrews or the British Red Cross (*see page 174*).

CONTENTS

WHAT TO DO IN AN EMERGENCY

WHEN TO CALL AN AMBULANCE

◆ IF YOU HAVE A HELPER, always send him to call an ambulance immediately.

◆ IF YOU ARE ALONE AND CASUALTY'S BREATHING IS ABSENT due to injury or drowning, resuscitate for one minute before calling an ambulance. For any other adult casualty, call an ambulance after noting that breathing is absent, then continue to resuscitate the casualty until help arrives.

◆ IF YOU ARE ALONE AND AN UNCONSCIOUS CASUALTY IS BREATHING, place him in the recovery position and then call an ambulance.

1 ASSESS THE CASUALTY (see opposite)

If he is conscious	If he is unconscious
Treat any injuries (see pages 153–60).	Go to step 2.

2 OPEN AIRWAY AND CHECK BREATHING (see opposite)

If he is breathing	If he is not breathing
Place him in the recovery position (see page 150).	Go to step 3.

3 GIVE MOUTH-TO-MOUTH VENTILATION (see page 151)

Go to step 4.

4 CHECK THE PULSE (see page 151)

If circulation is present	If circulation is absent
Continue mouth-to-mouth ventilation and keep checking the pulse.	Go to step 5.

5 GIVE CPR (see page 152)

Give a combination of chest compressions and mouth-to-mouth ventilation until help arrives.

UNCONSCIOUSNESS

I F A PERSON COLLAPSES in front of you, immediately establish whether or not he is conscious. If he is unconscious, you must open his airway, check whether or not he is breathing and, if necessary, begin resuscitation. For information on when to call an ambulance, see box opposite.

ASSESSING THE CASUALTY

1 **CHECK FOR CONSCIOUSNESS** Ask the casualty a question and gently shake his shoulders. If there is no response, the casualty is unconscious.

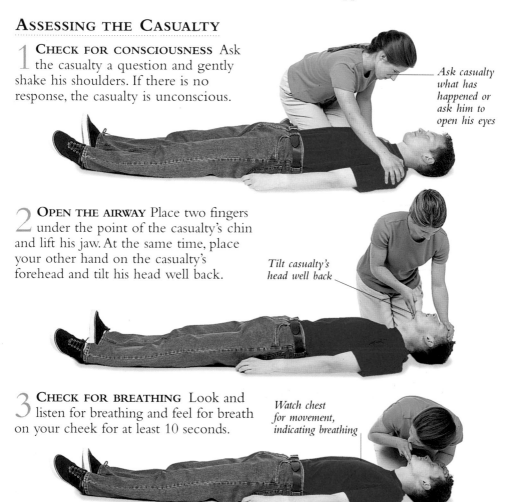

Ask casualty what has happened or ask him to open his eyes

2 **OPEN THE AIRWAY** Place two fingers under the point of the casualty's chin and lift his jaw. At the same time, place your other hand on the casualty's forehead and tilt his head well back.

Tilt casualty's head well back

3 **CHECK FOR BREATHING** Look and listen for breathing and feel for breath on your cheek for at least 10 seconds.

Watch chest for movement, indicating breathing

IF BREATHING IS PRESENT, place in the recovery position, *see overleaf* ▶
IF BREATHING IS ABSENT, give mouth-to-mouth ventilation, *see page 151* ▶

IF BREATHING IS PRESENT

IF THE CASUALTY IS BREATHING, he must be placed in the recovery position to stop his tongue from blocking his throat and to prevent him from inhaling vomit. If you suspect spinal injury, you *must* get a helper to support the casualty's head throughout the turn to keep the head and trunk aligned.

RECOVERY POSITION

1 **POSITION HAND** Tuck the hand nearest to you, arm straight and palm uppermost, under the casualty's thigh.

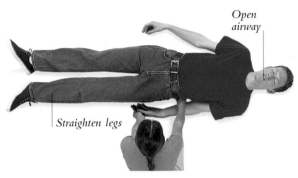

Open airway

Straighten legs

IF you suspect spinal injury, get help to turn casualty and maintain an open airway.

---

2 **PREPARE TO ROLL CASUALTY** Bring the arm furthest from you across the casualty's chest. Place his hand, palm outwards, against his cheek. With your other hand, pull up the knee furthest from you.

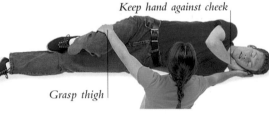

Keep hand against cheek

Grasp thigh

3 **ROLL CASUALTY TOWARDS YOU** Keeping his hand pressed against his cheek, pull at his thigh and roll him on to his side. Use your knees to support him and prevent him rolling forwards.

4 **MAKE ANY NECESSARY ADJUSTMENTS** Check the position of the casualty: his head should be tilted back; his hip and knee should be at right angles to his body; his lower arm should be free and lying along his back.

☎ **Call an ambulance.** Record breathing and pulse rate (*see page 161*).

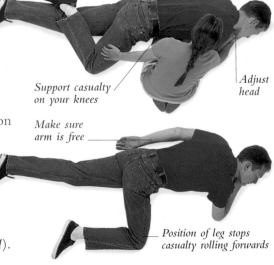

Support casualty on your knees

Adjust head

Make sure arm is free

Position of leg stops casualty rolling forwards

IF BREATHING IS ABSENT

I F A CASUALTY IS NOT BREATHING, you must give artificial ventilation. The most common form is mouth-to-mouth, but for a person who has had his voice box removed use the mouth-to-stoma technique (*see box below*).

MOUTH-TO-MOUTH VENTILATION

1 **REMOVE ANY OBSTRUCTION** Look into the casualty's mouth and remove any *obvious* obstruction.

2 **MAINTAIN OPEN AIRWAY** Keep two fingers under his chin and the other on his forehead, to tilt his head back.

3 **PINCH THE NOSE** Using your index finger and thumb of the hand that is resting on his forehead, pinch his nostrils tightly closed to prevent air escaping.

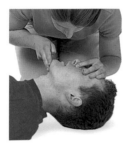

4 **BLOW INTO THE MOUTH** Take a full breath. Place your lips around the casualty's mouth. Make a good seal and blow into his mouth until the chest rises. Take two seconds for full inflation. Remove your lips, allow the chest to fall fully and repeat once.

MOUTH-TO-STOMA VENTILATION

If a person has had his voice box (*larynx*) removed, ventilation must be given through the opening in the front of the neck (*stoma*). If the person is a "partial neck breather", close off the mouth and nose with your fingers to prevent air escaping.

AFTER GIVING TWO VENTILATIONS, assess for circulation **see below** ▼

ASSESSING FOR CIRCULATION

C HECK THE PULSE. Use two fingers to feel for the pulse on the side of the neck. While you are doing this, look for any signs of recovery, such as return of colour to the skin and any movement.

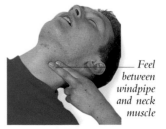

Feel between windpipe and neck muscle

DO NOT check the pulse for over 10 seconds.

IF CIRCULATION IS PRESENT, continue mouth-to-mouth **see above** ▶
IF CIRCULATION IS ABSENT, give cardiopulmonary resuscitation **see overleaf** ▶

IF CIRCULATION IS PRESENT

IF THE PULSE IS PRESENT, continue mouth-to-mouth ventilation. Check the pulse again and look for signs of recovery (*see page 151*) after every 10 breaths.
If at any time the pulse is absent, begin cardiopulmonary resuscitation immediately (*see below*).

IF CIRCULATION IS ABSENT

IF THERE IS NO PULSE or sign of recovery, you will have to provide an artificial circulation by giving cardiopulmonary resuscitation (CPR). This is a combination of chest compressions and artificial ventilations.

GIVING CPR

1 **POSITION YOUR FINGERS** Place the middle finger of your lower hand where the ribs meet the breastbone, and your index finger on the breastbone.

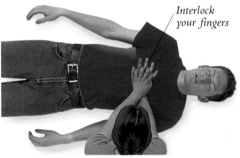

Interlock your fingers

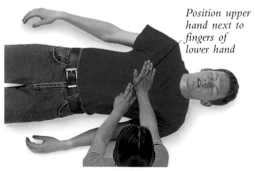

Position upper hand next to fingers of lower hand

2 **POSITION OTHER HAND** Place the heel of your other hand on the breastbone. Slide it down to your index finger and interlock your fingers.

3 **BEGIN CHEST COMPRESSIONS** Lean well over the casualty with your arms straight. Press down on the breastbone to depress it approximately 4–5cm (1½–2in). Complete 15 chest compressions, aiming for a rate of about 100 per minute.

4 **GIVE TWO BREATHS OF ARTIFICIAL VENTILATION** (*see page 151*) Continue alternating 15 compressions to 2 ventilations until help arrives.

HEART ATTACK

A HEART ATTACK most commonly occurs when the blood supply to part of the heart muscle is obstructed, for example, by a clot in one of the coronary arteries. Angina can be the body's way of warning of a heart attack and medical help should be sought. This condition occurs when narrowed arteries cannot deliver enough blood to meet the demands of exertion or excitement.

RECOGNITION
There may be: ◆ vice-like chest pain, starting at mid-chest and possibly radiating to the neck and the left arm; ◆ breathlessness and discomfort in the upper abdomen; ◆ sudden faintness or giddiness; ◆ ashen skin and blue lips; ◆ a rapid pulse, becoming weaker; ◆ collapse.

WHAT YOU SHOULD DO

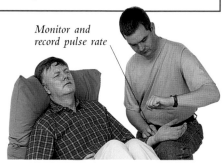

Monitor and record pulse rate

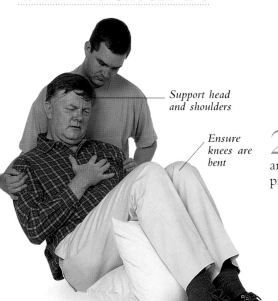

Support head and shoulders

Ensure knees are bent

1 MAKE THE CASUALTY COMFORTABLE A half-sitting position with knees bent is usually best.

☎ Call an ambulance. Tell the controller you suspect a heart attack.

2 MONITOR THE CASUALTY Check and record the casualty's breathing and pulse rate (*see page 161*). Be prepared to resuscitate (*see pages 151–52*).

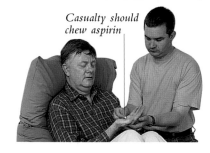

Casualty should chew aspirin

3 GIVE THE CASUALTY ONE ASPIRIN Tell him to chew, not swallow whole.

DO NOT give him any water.

CHOKING

IF A PERSON SWALLOWS FOOD that has been inadequately chewed and hurriedly swallowed, she may choke. This can block the throat or induce muscle spasms. Prompt action is required: you should be prepared to resuscitate (*see pages 151–52*).

RECOGNITION
There will be: ◆ difficulty speaking and breathing; ◆ initially, a congested face, and later, grey-blue skin; ◆ signs of distress, such as grasping the neck.

WHAT YOU SHOULD DO

IF the casualty becomes unconscious, or the obstruction does not clear after three cycles, place her in the recovery position and ☎ **call an ambulance**. Continue cycles.

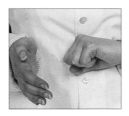

2 **POSITION HAND** Make a fist and position your hand with the thumb side against the abdomen.

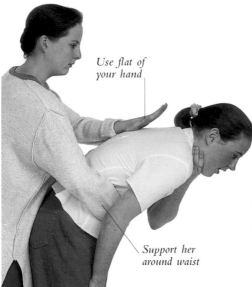

Use flat of your hand

Support her around waist

1 **GIVE FIVE BACK SLAPS** Bend the casualty well forwards and slap her firmly between the shoulder blades up to five times.

3 **GIVE ABDOMINAL THRUSTS** Grasp the fist with your other hand. Pull sharply inwards and upwards up to five times.

Position hands below ribcage

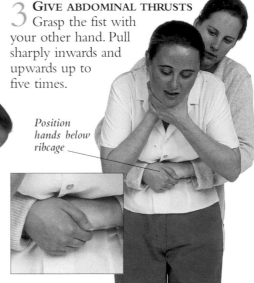

4 **REPEAT STEPS 1 TO 3** Continue with up to five back slaps and up to five abdominal thrusts alternately until the obstruction clears.

BURNS

WHEN TREATING BURNS that are deep or that extend over a large area, you must act quickly to cool the burn, relieve pain and minimise the extent of the injury. Your other priorities are to prevent infection occurring, check the casualty's breathing and be prepared to resuscitate her (see pages 151–52) if breathing is absent.

DO NOT remove any clothing or material that is sticking to the burned area.

DO NOT apply any lotions, ointments or fat.

DO NOT touch the burned area or burst any blisters.

DO NOT cover a facial burn.

WHAT YOU SHOULD DO

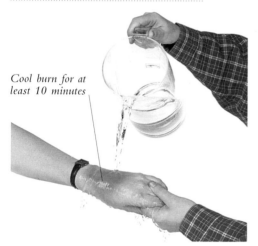

Cool burn for at least 10 minutes

1 DOUSE WITH COLD WATER
Thorough cooling of the burn may take at least 10 minutes, but must not delay removal to hospital.

2 MONITOR BREATHING
Watch for signs of difficulty in breathing while cooling the burn, and be prepared to resuscitate (see pages 151–52).

☎ **Call an ambulance.** Give the controller details of the injury.

3 REMOVE CLOTHING AND JEWELLERY
Remove these if they are on or around the burned area.

4 COVER THE WOUND
Use a sterile dressing to protect against infection.

IF a sterile dressing is not available, use a piece of clingfilm instead. Hold it by the edges as you apply it. Discard the first part of the roll and, once the film is applied, do not seal it.

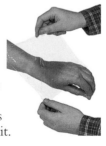

---

5 MONITOR THE CASUALTY
Stay with the casualty and treat her for shock (see page 160), if necessary.

SEVERE BLEEDING

SPURTING BLOOD, or severe bleeding that does not stop within five minutes, can be life-threatening. You must take action to stop the bleeding immediately. Be prepared to resuscitate the casualty if she loses consciousness (*see pages 151–52*) and treat her for shock (*see page 160*), if necessary.

WHAT YOU SHOULD DO

1 **EXPOSE WOUND** Wearing gloves, if you have a pair to hand, remove or cut clothing from the injured area.

2 **APPLY DIRECT PRESSURE** Preferably using a clean pad or sterile dressing, press the wound for 10 minutes to give the blood time to clot.

3 **RAISE THE INJURED LIMB** Support it above the level of the casualty's heart.

4 **LAY CASUALTY DOWN** This will reduce the blood flow to the site of the injury and minimise the shock caused.

Keep limb raised

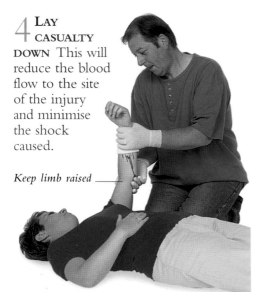

5 **APPLY A DRESSING OR BANDAGE** Leave any original pad in place. If any blood seeps through, apply an additional dressing.

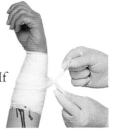

DO NOT bandage too tightly.

IF there is an object protruding from the wound, build up padding on either side of it, until it is possible to bandage over it without applying any pressure.

☎ **Call an ambulance.** Explain the severity of the injury to the controller.

6 **MONITOR CASUALTY** Check and record breathing, pulse rate and level of response (*see page 161*). Treat for shock (*see page 160*), if necessary.

HYPOTHERMIA

PEOPLE WHO ARE immobile, frail or ill (particularly the elderly) are susceptible to hypothermia. This condition develops when the body temperature falls below 35°C (95°F). An elderly person's body loses its sensitivity to cold so she may not be aware of a drop in her body temperature. Lack of agility, chronic illness and fatigue can all increase the risk of hypothermia, as can a poorly heated home. If the correct preventive measures are taken (*see page 129*), there is no reason why indoor hypothermia should occur.

RECOGNITION
There may be: ◆ temperature of below 35°C (95°F); ◆ slow, weakening pulse; ◆ shivering, and cold, pale, dry skin; ◆ lethargy; ◆ slow, shallow breathing; ◆ apathy, disorientation, irrational behaviour.

WHAT YOU SHOULD DO

1 **REWARM GRADUALLY** Cover an elderly casualty with layers of blankets in a room temperature of approximately 25°C (77°F).

DO NOT allow an elderly person to have a bath or use direct heat sources, such as hot-water bottles or fires, for rewarming.

2 **PROVIDE WARM DRINKS** Soup or high-energy foods, such as chocolate, will help.

☎ **Call a doctor.** You must always get medical assistance if the casualty is elderly, as hypothermia may disguise the symptoms of a stroke or heart attack.

DO NOT give the casualty any alcohol.

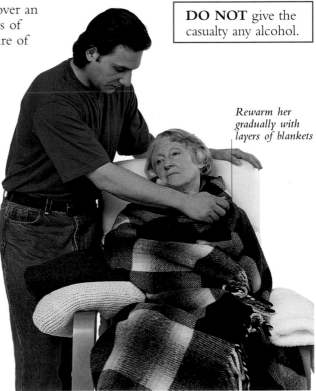

Rewarm her gradually with layers of blankets

STROKE

THIS OCCURS WHEN the blood supply to the brain is suddenly impaired by a clot or ruptured blood vessels. Strokes are more common in later life, especially in those with high blood pressure or a circulatory disorder. The effect of the stroke depends on how much, and which part, of the brain is affected. Major strokes can be fatal, but many people make a complete recovery from minor ones. For an unconscious casualty who has suffered a stroke, your main aims are to get urgent medical help and, if needed, begin resuscitation (*see pages 151–52*).

RECOGNITION
There may be: ◆ sudden, severe headache; ◆ sudden or gradual loss of consciousness; ◆ dribbling mouth and slurred speech; ◆ loss of power or movement in limbs; ◆ pupils of unequal size; ◆ loss of bladder or bowel control; ◆ a confused, emotional state.

WHAT YOU SHOULD DO

FOR AN UNCONSCIOUS CASUALTY

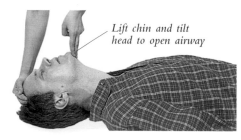

Lift chin and tilt head to open airway

1 **FOLLOW RESUSCITATION PROCEDURE** (*see page 148*) Open the airway, check breathing and circulation. If breathing, place in recovery position.

2 **LOOSEN ANY CLOTHING** Undo anything that may impede breathing.

☎ **Call an ambulance.** Tell the controller that you suspect a stroke.

3 **MONITOR CASUALTY** Check and record the breathing and pulse rate (*see page 161*) until help arrives.

FOR A CONSCIOUS CASUALTY

DO NOT give the casualty any food or drink.

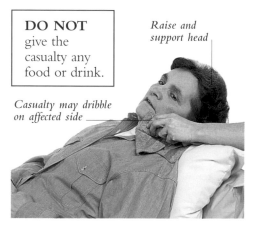

Raise and support head

Casualty may dribble on affected side

1 **LAY THE CASUALTY DOWN** Position the casualty with her head and shoulders slightly raised and supported.

2 **INCLINE HER HEAD TO ONE SIDE** Place a towel or cloth on her shoulder to absorb any dribbling.

☎ **Call an ambulance.** Tell the controller that you suspect a stroke.

BROKEN BONES

BONES CAN BE WEAKENED by age or disease, which makes them more susceptible to breaking or crumbling. Always remember to move elderly people carefully, even if there is no history of violent injury or broken bones. For an open fracture, always stop any severe bleeding first.

RECOGNITION

For a closed fracture there will be:
◆ bruising and swelling at the fracture site;
◆ severe pain around the injured area.
For an open fracture there will be:
◆ broken skin over the fracture site;
◆ an exposed bone and bleeding.

WHAT YOU SHOULD DO

1 **SUPPORT AFFECTED LIMB** Place your hands above and below the injury for support.

DO NOT move the limb unnecessarily.

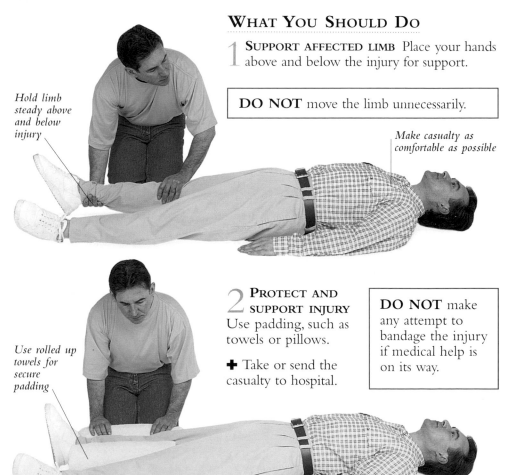

Hold limb steady above and below injury

Make casualty as comfortable as possible

2 **PROTECT AND SUPPORT INJURY** Use padding, such as towels or pillows.

✚ Take or send the casualty to hospital.

DO NOT make any attempt to bandage the injury if medical help is on its way.

Use rolled up towels for secure padding

SHOCK

THIS CONDITION DEVELOPS if the heart fails to pump blood around the circulatory system. It also occurs if blood supply to the vital organs is lost, through severe bleeding or fluid loss. Your aims are to treat any causes of the shock, especially severe bleeding, and ensure that the casualty is comfortable. Do not confuse circulatory shock with deep emotional stress.

RECOGNITION

At first there may be:
◆ a rapid pulse, becoming weaker;
◆ pale, grey skin, especially inside the lips;
◆ sweating and cold, clammy skin.

Later there may be:
◆ nausea and possible vomiting;
◆ weakness and giddiness;
◆ rapid, shallow breathing;
◆ thirst.

WHAT YOU SHOULD DO

1 **TREAT ANY CAUSE OF SHOCK**
Act quickly to treat any injuries.

2 **POSITION THE CASUALTY** Lay her down, preferably on a blanket, but without a pillow. Raise her legs and support them.

Raise legs to improve blood supply to heart

Lay her on her back

Keep head low

3 **LOOSEN ANY TIGHT CLOTHING**
Undo clothing, such as a belt, tie or tight collar, that may impede breathing.

DO NOT use direct heat to rewarm.

☎ Call an ambulance.

4 **MONITOR CASUALTY** Check and record breathing, pulse rate and level of response (*see opposite*). Be prepared to resuscitate, if needed (*see pages 151–52*).

Cover her with blanket for warmth

OBSERVATION CHART

ONCE YOU HAVE SUMMONED MEDICAL HELP, it is important to monitor the casualty. Make your own copies of the observation chart (*below*) and use one to record your findings, noting the casualty's pulse, breathing and level of response every 10 minutes, or more frequently for a critical casualty. The chart should then be passed to the medical services, where the information can be used to make decisions about how to treat the casualty.

DATE .... **CASUALTY'S NAME** ....

		Time (*10-minute intervals*)					
		10	20	30	40	50	60
Eyes Observe for reaction while testing other responses.	Open spontaneously						
	Open to speech						
	Open to painful stimulus						
	No response						
Movement Apply painful stimulus: pinch skin on back of hand, or ear lobe.	Obeys commands						
	Responds to painful stimulus						
	No response						
Speech When testing responses, speak clearly and directly, close to casualty's ear.	Responds sensibly to questions						
	Seems confused						
	Uses inappropriate words						
	Incomprehensible sounds						
	No response						
Pulse (beats per minute) Take pulse at wrist on conscious casualty (*see page 128*); At neck on unconscious casualty (*see page 151*); Note rate, if beats are weak (*w*) or strong (*s*), regular (*reg*) or irregular (*irreg*).	111–120						
	101–110						
	91–100						
	81–90						
	71–80						
	61–70						
	Below 60						
Breathing (breaths per minute) Note rate (*see page 128*), and whether breathing is quiet (*q*) or noisy (*n*), easy (*e*) or difficult (*diff*).	41–50						
	31–40						
	21–30						
	11–20						
	Below 10						

FIRST-AID MATERIALS

K EEP ALL YOUR FIRST-AID MATERIALS together in a container and keep the kit in a dry place. Check and replenish it regularly, so that you always have what you need to hand. The types and quantities of dressings and bandages required for a standard kit are shown below, as well as other useful items.

USEFUL DRESSINGS AND BANDAGES

20 assorted adhesive dressings
Use these for minor wounds. The waterproof variety is best for wounds on the hands.

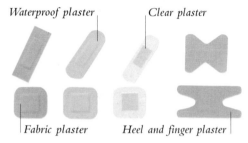

Waterproof plaster *Clear plaster*

Fabric plaster *Heel and finger plaster*

10 sterile dressings
These come in a range of sizes. Ideally, you should keep two large, two extra-large and six medium dressings.

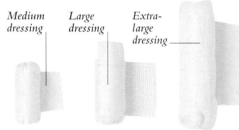

Medium dressing *Large dressing* *Extra-large dressing*

2 sterile eye pads
Any injury to the eye needs a sterile covering. Either type shown below will suffice.

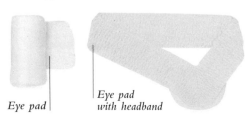

Eye pad *Eye pad with headband*

6 triangular bandages
These are made of strong paper or cloth. They can be used as bandages, slings or, if they are sterile and individually wrapped, as dressings.

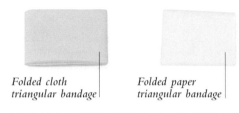

Folded cloth triangular bandage *Folded paper triangular bandage*

OTHER USEFUL ITEMS

In addition to the standard dressings and bandages, the items shown below are useful.

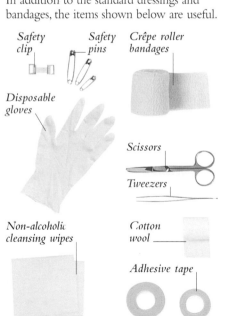

Safety clip *Safety pins* *Crêpe roller bandages*

Disposable gloves

Scissors

Tweezers

Non-alcoholic cleansing wipes *Cotton wool*

Adhesive tape

CHAPTER 15

USEFUL INFORMATION

The pages that follow aim to provide
all the information you need to maximise the benefits and
resources that may be available to you and your relative.

FINANCIAL INFORMATION

The financial section gives details of a range of
benefits to which you and your relative may be entitled. It
explains the procedure for applying for benefits and what to
do if your claim is turned down.

YOUR RIGHTS

The Carers Act was passed to protect the rights of carers, and to
ensure that proper assessments are carried out. The Patient's
Charter aims to make patients aware of their right to proper
medical care and treatment. Both documents are summarised here.

USEFUL ADDRESSES

As well as the help and support provided by your
local authority, you may benefit from the advice of specialist
organisations. This section gives addresses and telephone numbers
for a range of organisations that can offer advice and practical and
emotional support to you and/or your relative.

Claiming Benefits

MANY CARERS DO NOT CLAIM BENEFITS because they are unsure who to contact and/or are put off by the application procedure. With a little preparation, however, making a claim should be quite straightforward. You just need to be clear about what you require, have as much information to hand as possible and be patient, but persistent.

Do's & Don'ts

☑ **Do** apply for benefits, even if you are not sure that you qualify.

☑ **Do** seek advice, either directly from the Benefits Agency or from an advice centre (*see page 167*), as the system for claiming benefits can be confusing and there are often set rules and procedures to follow.

☒ **Don't** delay in applying. Many benefits are payable from the date of application and cannot be backdated.

☒ **Don't** be intimidated by the forms or by complicated procedures. Seek advice rather than not bothering to apply.

☒ **Don't** feel ashamed or embarrassed about making a claim. If you do not claim a benefit, you and your relative could lose out on money specifically allocated by the government for helping elderly, ill or disabled people.

Applying for Benefits

If you think you or your relative are entitled to benefits, contact the Benefits Agency by telephoning the freephone helpline (*see page 177*). Ask the agency what benefits you may be entitled to and ask them to send you the relevant application forms. Your application will be assessed by an adjudicating officer (AO), who is obliged to reply to you within 14 days.

Organisation tips

Try to be prepared and organised.

Obtain advance information Before you contact the Benefits Agency, find out your rights from an organisation such as the Citizens Advice Bureau.

Prepare your questions Make a checklist of questions in advance so that you don't forget anything.

Fill in forms carefully Fill forms in as promptly and accurately as possible. Seek advice (*see page 167*) or telephone the helpline if anything is unclear.

Keep a record Take copies of all correspondence and keep a record of telephone conversations.

Information You Need

Before a proper assessment can be made, you will be required to supply information about yourself and your relative, both verbally and on forms. Try to prepare some of the information in advance, such as:

- details of your income and savings;
- dates of birth;
- mortgage or rent details;
- National Insurance numbers;
- previous correspondence about benefits;
- a doctor's note (this may be required for some benefits).

TYPES OF BENEFITS

T HERE IS A RANGE OF BENEFITS outlined here and on the following pages, together with the criteria needed to qualify. You can also obtain explanatory leaflets from the Benefits Agency. You will find that claiming one benefit may affect your right to claim for others. The information on page 168 is a quick reference guide to how the benefits are grouped.

INVALID CARE ALLOWANCE (ICA)

This is the main benefit available for carers. It is an earnings replacement benefit because, as a carer, you will be unable to fulfil your earnings potential. To claim this allowance, you do not have to live with or be related to the person in your care.

HOW TO QUALIFY
♦ You must be of working age (between 16 and 65).
♦ You must be a carer for at least 35 hours a week – this time does not have to be spread evenly throughout the week.
♦ The person you are caring for must be receiving either the Attendance Allowance, Constant Attendance Allowance or the middle or higher part of the Disability Living Allowance (*see overleaf*).
♦ You must be a resident in Great Britain (special rules apply to the armed forces).

RESTRICTIONS
♦ If there is more than one carer, only one can apply.
♦ If you are caring for two people, you can only receive one allowance.
♦ If you do work for part of the week, you must earn less than a given amount.
♦ If your relative also receives benefits, these may be affected; seek advice before making a claim.
♦ You lose the benefit immediately if the person in your care dies or no longer needs your assistance.

ADVANTAGES OF CLAIMING
♦ If you pay an outside carer when you do work, this will be taken into account when assessing your income.
♦ Your pension will not be affected.
♦ You can backdate your claim by up to three months.

THE CARER PREMIUM

The Carer Premium (CP) is only paid to carers who qualify for Invalid Care Allowance (ICA) and is paid as part of Income Support, Housing Benefit or Council Tax Rebate. If you are granted ICA, the ICA unit will tell your Benefits Agency office, who will pay CP with your Income Support. If you are already getting Housing Benefit or Council Tax Rebate, then tell your benefit office that you have been awarded ICA and your benefit will be recalculated accordingly.

If you stop being a carer CP will be paid for a further eight weeks after you stop, during which time you do not have to sign on as unemployed. If you have a problem, ring your local Citizens Advice Bureau or the Benefits Agency freephone helpline (*see page 177*).

DISABILITY BENEFITS FOR YOUR RELATIVE

TYPE OF BENEFIT	HOW TO QUALIFY	NOTES
Incapacity Benefit	◆ The person must be unable to work as a result of sickness or disability. ◆ National Insurance must have been paid.	◆ This allowance reduces Income Support, but may lead to an increase in other benefits. ◆ The rate paid is related to the period of illness.
Severe Disablement Allowance	◆ The person must be severely disabled or have become disabled before the age of 20. ◆ The person must never have worked or never have paid National Insurance.	◆ This differs from the Incapacity Benefit because it does not depend on the amount of National Insurance that has been paid.
Disability Living Allowance	◆ The person must be disabled and under 65. ◆ The person must need personal care or supervision for at least three months (unless terminally ill). This is the care component. ◆ The person must be severely immobile and need someone to act as a guide. This is the mobility component.	◆ There are different levels of payment for the mobility and care components of the allowance, depending on the severity of the person's needs. It is possible for a person to receive both parts. ◆ Eligibility can lead to payment of extra benefits.
Attendance Allowance	◆ The person must be disabled and under 65. ◆ The person must need help with personal care, such as washing and dressing.	◆ Unlike the Disability Living Allowance, this does not provide help for mobility needs.
Disability Working Allowance	◆ The person must be disabled and working. ◆ The person must receive a low income.	◆ This may not be awarded if savings are above a certain amount.
Constant Attendance Allowance	◆ The person must receive Industrial Injury Benefit or a War Pension and need constant care.	◆ Care needs are defined in the same way as for the Disability Living Allowance.

GENERAL BENEFITS

There is a range of other benefits for which you and your relative may be eligible, either because you have a low income or because you are unable to work. Your savings will also be taken into consideration.

INCOME SUPPORT

This depends on your savings and income; if you receive this you are eligible for other health benefits.

FAMILY CREDIT

This benefit is aimed at families on a low income with dependants.

COUNCIL TAX REBATE

This depends on your income and savings; carers may be entitled to additional council tax reductions.

HOUSING BENEFIT

This is awarded if you pay rent and are on a low income; if you receive Invalid Care Allowance you may be assessed on a more generous scale.

HEALTH BENEFITS

This subsidises health needs, such as dental and eye care. It is assessed on your income and savings.

SOCIAL FUND

A range of grants and loans is available for people on low incomes to help with essentials, such as bedding.

IF AN APPLICATION IS REJECTED

If your application is rejected, you can almost always appeal. The adjudicating officer is legally obliged to explain in writing why your application was turned down, and if you do not agree with the reasons given, you can make an appeal; this is why it is important to keep a record of all correspondence. Different benefits have different time limits within which you can make an appeal, so the sooner you question a decision the better. It is advisable to seek professional help before making an appeal. Try contacting your local Citizens Advice Bureau or The Law Society (*see page 177*).

ADVICE CENTRES

The various benefits and your entitlements can be confusing. There are centres with specially trained staff that advise on a range of issues, including benefits. These centres include:
- Citizens Advice Bureaux;
- Welfare Rights Centres;
- Independent Advice Centres.

The telephone numbers of these organisations may be listed in your local telephone directory or Yellow Pages; if not, your local library or council office should be able to direct you.

Going to a centre
Some advice centres have open sessions where you can see an adviser (usually for no longer than 15 minutes) without making an appointment. However, this may involve a long wait. If this is not practical for you, for example, because you cannot leave your relative unattended, ask for a meeting by ringing the centre or making a request in writing. If you cannot leave your relative alone, it may be possible for a representative to visit you at home.

COMBINING BENEFITS

RECEIVING ONE TYPE OF BENEFIT may restrict you and your relative from claiming another benefit or affect the amount received. It is also easy to overlook a benefit to which you may be entitled. It is important that you claim the right combination of benefits, as the information below outlines, otherwise you may be losing out on money that is rightfully yours.

COMBINATIONS OF BENEFITS THAT CAN BE CLAIMED

You can usually claim one benefit or allowance from each of the groups listed below. For example, someone claiming Disability Living Allowance cannot claim Attendance Allowance as well. Eligibility may also depend on National Insurance contributions.

One of Group 1:
- **Invalid Care Allowance** (*see page 165*)
- **Incapacity Benefit** (*see page 166*)
- **Severe Disablement Allowance** (*see page 166*)
- **Widow's Pension** Paid to women who were aged 45 and over when widowed.
- **Widowed Mother's Allowance** Paid to women who were widowed with a dependent child or while pregnant.
- **State Retirement Pension** Paid to women aged 60 or over and men aged 65 or over.
- **Job Seeker's Allowance** (Unemployment Benefit) Paid to those available and actively looking for work.
- **Maternity Allowance** Paid to pregnant women who have recently worked.

Plus either or both of Group 2:
- **Industrial Injuries Benefit** Paid to those who become sick or disabled as a result of their work.

- **War Pension** Paid to those who become sick or disabled during or after service in the armed forces.

Plus one of Group 3:
- **Disability Living Allowance** (*see page 166*)
- **Attendance Allowance** (*see page 166*)
- **Constant Attendance Allowance** (*see page 166*)

Plus one of Group 4:
- **Income Support** (*see page 167*)
- **Family Credit** (*see page 167*)
- **Disability Working Allowance** (*see page 166*)

Plus any of Group 5:
- **Housing Benefit** (*see page 167*)
- **Council Tax Rebate** (*see page 167*)
- **Health Benefits** (*see page 167*)
- **Social Fund** (*see page 167*)
- **Child Benefit** Paid to a parent with a dependent child.
- **One Parent Benefit** Paid to a parent bringing up a child on his own.
- **Guardian's Allowance** Paid to a person looking after someone else's child.

Plus Group 6:
- **National Insurance Credits** Paid to maintain National Insurance contributions, which may be affected if you are receiving benefits.

MANAGING MONEY

I F YOU ARE LOOKING AFTER YOUR RELATIVE, and perhaps other dependants, you may find that you have to balance high outgoings with a low income (especially if you have given up your job). To stay financially stable, you need to minimise your outgoings by working out how you can spend less, and maximise your income, not least by exploring your options for financial help.

BUDGETING EFFICIENTLY

To keep your finances in order, it is advisable to work out a weekly or monthly budget. If you are constantly over budget or short of money for essential items such as food, clothing and bills, you need to look carefully at your income and outgoings to establish whether you need help.

ASSESSING YOUR INCOME AND OUTGOINGS

Consider the questions below to work out where you could save money or where help may be available.

◆ Are you and your relative receiving your full entitlement of benefits? Look at the information on pages 164–68 and seek advice, if necessary.

◆ Can you get any help with bills? Utility companies, for example, gas and electricity, often have special facilities for helping people who cannot make a payment. There are also charities that help people who are struggling to pay bills.

◆ Are you spending money on items for which you could be receiving subsidies, such as prescription charges or dental care?

◆ Are you spreading your bills evenly over the year? Smaller monthly bills are often easier to handle than big quarterly demands. Look into setting up a direct debit with your bank or building society, save through a budget scheme or buy savings stamps.

◆ Could others in your household be contributing more? Perhaps you have children living with you who are earning, but don't pay rent. Ask if they could contribute in small ways, such as taking it in turns to pay the telephone bill or the weekly food bill.

◆ As a last resort, is there any part-time work you could do from home? This could just be on a temporary basis until you are more financially stable.

DO'S & DON'TS

If you get into debt, do not panic; there is always a way out if you seek help early enough.

✓ **Do** seek advice. Organisations, such as the Citizens Advice Bureau (*see page 177*), may be able to help you find a way of repaying your debts. Give details of all your debts, however huge they may be.

✓ **Do** prioritise your debts. For example, it is more essential to pay a utilities bill to prevent your supplies being cut off, than to pay your credit card bill.

✓ **Don't** be embarrassed to ask for help. Advisers will not be judgemental.

✗ **Don't** just ignore the debt. This will not make it go away.

✗ **Don't** take out one loan to pay for another. It may solve the problem temporarily, but it will only plunge you deeper into debt in the end.

COURT OF PROTECTION

If you do not have an Enduring Power of Attorney and your relative becomes mentally ill, you will be unable to access money that could be used for him, such as his savings or pension. In this situation you can apply in writing to the Court of Protection (*see page 177*). The court then supervises the management of your relative's affairs, and charges an income-related fee for this.

Low income If your relative's income is not very high, the court will allow you to use his money without having to refer to the court again.

A receiver If your relative's assets are in excess of £5000, the court will appoint a receiver, usually a close relative or friend, but in some situations a bank manager or solicitor, to manage your relative's affairs. The court must then supervise the receiver, asking to see a record of all receipts and payments made by him on behalf of your relative. This protects your relative's affairs and ensures they are being properly managed.

MANAGING SOMEONE'S FINANCES

You may have to oversee your relative's financial affairs if he is unable to manage them himself. How this is done will depend entirely on his condition – that is, whether he is physically or mentally impaired – and his financial status. You should both seek independent advice from a solicitor or advice centre (*see page 167*) before making any arrangements.

BECOMING AN AGENT OR APPOINTEE

If your relative's only income is Social Security benefit and he is mentally capable but physically unable to leave his home, you may need to become his Agent. This means that you cash his order book on his behalf, while he retains responsibility for filling in claim forms and reporting any changes in his circumstances. If your relative is mentally ill, you could become an Appointee: this gives you full responsibility for the account, rather than just cashing in the allowance. It also means that you must report any changes in circumstances. Being an Appointee also means that you are responsible for repaying any debts.

OPENING A JOINT ACCOUNT

This will allow you to withdraw money for your relative's needs whenever they arise. This can be done with either a bank or building society account.

THIRD PARTY MANDATE

Instead of opening a joint account, your relative can give you a Third Party Mandate to operate his account. He simply writes a letter to his bank or building society requesting the mandate. Most establishments have a standard letter prepared.

POWER OF ATTORNEY

A Power of Attorney gives you legal control of your relative's money, but it becomes invalid if your relative becomes mentally ill. An Enduring Power of Attorney gives you greater rights over his affairs because it enables you to continue managing your relative's finances, even if he becomes mentally ill. However, this right has to be granted to you before your relative has become mentally incapable.

MAKING A WILL

O NE OF THE MOST ESSENTIAL ARRANGEMENTS to be made by you and your relative is a will. This is a legal document that enables a person to leave his money, property and possessions to those who are important to him. If a person dies without leaving a will, the law decides how the property should be divided up and this may exclude those he wishes to provide for.

MAKING A WILL

It is possible for you and your relative to write a will yourselves but, if it is unclear in any way, there is a risk that your wishes may not be carried out. It is advisable, therefore, to employ a solicitor or will-writing specialist, who will require you to supply the following information:
◆ a list detailing the value of any property and possessions (the estate), including everything from mortgage details to the value of the silverware;
◆ the people (executors) that are appointed to take charge of the estate. This could be a solicitor or accountant (who will charge), but a friend or relative may also be chosen;
◆ details of the people or institutions that are to inherit (the beneficiaries), specifying exactly what is to be left and to whom;
◆ the value of any debts. Note that a beneficiary will have to repay the debt on mortgaged property unless otherwise specified;
◆ name(s) of any guardian(s) that are appointed to look after children.

IF THERE IS NO WILL

If you are dependent on the person you are caring for (for example, he owns the house that you live in) and he has not made a will, you may feel anxious about your future. You can raise the subject tactfully, but you cannot force him to make a will or amend it to include you. It may be that he does not feel ready to make a will because he is unable to accept his impending death; he may see making a will as a sign of giving up, or he may just be too mentally frail to understand. A solicitor or local Citizens Advice Bureau will be able to advise you of your rights.

TAX IMPLICATIONS AFTER DEATH

After someone dies you may get tax allowances or have to pay tax on inherited goods.

Tax allowances If your spouse dies, you are entitled to a number of tax allowances for the year in which he dies and the following year. Ask your local tax office for more information, or ask for a tax guide at your local library.

Inheritance Tax When a person dies his estate is subject to Inheritance Tax if its value is above a certain level. Even if the person's money and possessions do not amount to a great deal, the value of his property could be higher than you realise and could be enough to make the overall value of the estate subject to the tax. Foresight and careful wording of a will could save beneficiaries thousands of pounds.

THE CARERS ACT

IF YOU ARE LOOKING AFTER SOMEONE who has an illness or disability, regardless of that person's age, relationship to you or whether or not you live with them, you are a carer. As a carer, you may be entitled to help from Social Services. The Carers Recognition and Services Act (1995) – or Carers Act – aims to give carers a voice and helps them to get assistance.

THE AIM OF THE ACT

Social Services is obliged under the NHS and Community Care Act (1990) to assess and provide care to sick and disabled people who wish to continue living at home. Before any help can be given, that person and anyone involved in caring for her, has a right to be assessed by a social worker, appointed by Social Services. If necessary, the assessor will call in specialists, such as a doctor or nurse, to give advice about the person's requirements.

THE ASSESSMENT

At the assessment you should make sure that any problems are raised. Make a list in advance of everything you need to discuss, such as any day-to-day problems your relative has – she may, for example, have difficulty climbing stairs – and any aspects of caring you are finding difficult – you may, for example, need help with turning your relative during the night.

HELP ON OFFER

Social Services can help in different ways. They may provide direct care in the form of home helps, voluntary carers or residential homes, or may assist you to give care by arranging and funding adaptations to your home or by providing specialist equipment so that your relative can be more independent.

WHO PAYS?

An assessment under the Carer's Act is free, but the services provided may not be. As these services are for your relative, she will be asked questions about her finances. Charges may vary from area to area but, by law, Social Services cannot ask a person to contribute more than she can reasonably afford. Sometimes local authorities make cash payments to the person in care, in lieu of directly providing a service. For example, if your relative needs a home help, the local authority may contribute so you or your relative can employ someone directly. However, if a local authority has limited funds, it is legally entitled to withhold or withdraw help. So, although you and the person you are caring for do have the right to be assessed, you may not always get the help you need.

MAKING A COMPLAINT

If you or your relative are not satisfied with the outcome of your assessment, you can complain, ideally in writing, to Social Services. The matter should then be referred to an independent panel for review. Your local Citizens Advice Bureau (*see page 177*) may be able to help and advise you about the complaints procedure.

THE PATIENT'S CHARTER

EVERY PATIENT HAS THE RIGHT to expect a certain standard of care from the National Health Service (NHS). The Patient's Charter sets out exactly what these standards are and outlines standards that the NHS aims to achieve. If your relative is denied a service or treated inappropriately, it is important that she knows when she is within her right to complain.

THE AIM OF THE CHARTER

The Patient's Charter outlines the rights of an NHS patient and aims to set levels in standards of care. It details the type of treatment and care the patient has a *right* to receive and outlines what a patient can *expect* to receive, although it may not always be possible to provide the latter. It legally binds the NHS to provide services set out in the Charter to the agreed standards. Consequently, if a patient receives medical care or a service that falls below the set standard, she can lodge a complaint.

THE PATIENT'S RIGHTS

These are some of a patient's basic rights under the Patient's Charter:
◆ to receive healthcare based on medical need for it, not on ability to pay;
◆ to have the risks involved in any treatment explained to you, and be told what the alternatives are, before agreeing to accept it;
◆ to obtain emergency medical treatment at any time;
◆ to be referred to a consultant when the GP thinks it necessary and to be referred for a second opinion (if the GP agrees);
◆ to change GP quickly and easily;
◆ to have any complaint about an NHS service investigated;
◆ to choose whether or not to be involved in medical research.

WHAT A PATIENT CAN EXPECT

The Charter sets out standards of service that the NHS aims to provide but which at times may be impossible to meet. The NHS asserts that it is only in exceptional circumstances that these standards will not be met. For example:
◆ a patient can expect her privacy, dignity and religious and cultural beliefs to be respected at all times.
◆ before a patient is discharged from hospital, she can expect a decision to have been made about how she will be cared for once she is at home. The patient, and her carer, can expect to be involved in making the decisions and to be kept up-to-date with information at all stages.
◆ if a patient needs a home visit from a healthcare professional, such as a district nurse, she can expect to be consulted about a convenient time and expect a visit within two hours of the stated time.

FURTHER INFORMATION

The Patient's Charter is fully explained in a free booklet entitled *The Patient's Charter and You*, available in English, eleven other languages, Braille, audio cassette and as a sign language video. This can be obtained by writing to:
THE PATIENT'S CHARTER
FREEPOST, NEA 959
WETHERBY LS23 6YY.

USEFUL ADDRESSES

VOLUNTARY AID SOCIETIES

St. John Ambulance
1 Grosvenor Crescent
London SW1X 7EF
0171 235 5231
(See page 12)

St. Andrew's Ambulance Association
St Andrew's House
Milton Street
Glasgow G4 0HR
0141 332 4031
(See page 12)

British Red Cross
9 Grosvenor Crescent
London SW1X 7EJ
0171 235 5454
(See page 12)

GENERAL SUPPORT GROUPS

Carers National Association
Ruth Pitter House
20–25 Glasshouse Yard
London EC1A 4JS
0171 490 8818
Carers line: 0345 573369
(Mon-Fri 10.00–12.00 and
14.00–16.00)
Scotland:
3rd Floor
162 Buchanan Street
Glasgow G1 2LL
0141 333 9455
Advises on all aspects of caring.

Crossroads Care Attendants Schemes
10 Regent Place
Rugby
Warwickshire CV21 2PN
01788 573653

Scotland:
24 George Square
Glasgow G2 1EG
0141 226 3793
Wales:
Ground Floor
Unit 5, Coopers Yard
Curran Road
Cardiff CF1 5DF
01222 222282

Provide trained care attendants as
part of a sitting service.

Counsel and Care
Lower Ground Floor
Twyman House
16 Bonny Street
London NW1 9PG
0171 485 1556
Advice: 0171 485 1566
(10.30–16.00)
Provides information for people over
pensionable age, including advice
about residential care.

Holiday Care Service
2nd Floor
Imperial Building
Victoria Road
Horley
Surrey RH6 7PZ
01293 774 535
Advises on holidays for disabled
people and carers.

Relatives Association
5 Tavistock Place
London WC1H 9SN
0171 916 6055
Provides advice for relatives and
friends of older people in residential
care and nursing homes.

Royal British Legion
48 Pall Mall
London SW1Y 5JY
0171 973 7200
Provides advice and support for
the ex-service community and
their dependants.

SSAFA Forces Help
Queen Elizabeth The Queen
Mother House
19 Queen Elizabeth Street
London SE1 2LP
0171 403 8783 or
0171 962 9696
A national charity that helps
serving and ex-service men, women
and their families in need.

ORGANISATIONS FOR SPECIFIC CONDITIONS

There are numerous organisations
that offer help and advice to sufferers
from specific conditions, and their
families.

AIDS CARE
Terrence Higgins Trust
52–54 Grays Inn Road
London WC1X 8JU
0171 831 0330

London Lighthouse
111–117 Lancaster Road
London W11 1QT
0171 792 1200

ALZHEIMER'S DISEASE
Alzheimer's Disease Society
Gordon House
10 Greencoat Place
London SW1P 1PH
0171 306 0606
Scotland:
Action on Dementia
22 Drumsheugh Gardens
Edinburgh EH3 7RN
0131 243 1453

ARTHRITIS
Arthritis Care
18 Stephenson Way
London NW1 3HD
0171 916 1500
Freephone Helpline:
0800 289 170

AUTISM
National Autistic Society
393 City Road
London EC1V 1NE
0171 833 2299

BACK PAIN
National Back Pain Association
16 Elmtree Road
Teddington
Middlesex TW11 8ST
0181 977 5474

BLINDNESS/VISUAL IMPAIRMENT
RNIB – Royal National Institute for the Blind
224 Great Portland Street
London W1N 6AA
0171 388 1266

Scotland:
10 Magdala Crescent
Edinburgh EH12 5BE
0131 313 1498

9 Clairmont Gardens
Glasgow G3 7LW
0141 332 0343

CANCER
BACUP – British Association of Cancer United Patients
3 Bath Place
Rivington Street
London EC2A 3JR
0171 696 9003

Scotland:
Counselling Service:
0141 553 1553

Cancer Information Service:
0171 613 2121
(*Mon-Fri 9.00-19.00*)
Cancer Information Service
from outside London:
0800 181 199
London-based
Counselling Service:
0171 696 9000

Cancerlink
17 Britannia Street
London WC1X 9JN
Tel & Text line
(*use voice announcer*):
0171 833 2451
Bengali & Hindi
0171 713 7867

Cancer Relief Macmillan Fund
Anchor House
15-19 Britten Street
London, SW3 3TZ
0171 351 7811

Scotland:
9 Castle Terrace
Edinburgh EH1 2DP
0131 229 3276
Provides information about Macmillan nurses for cancer care.

Marie Curie Cancer Care
28 Belgrave Square
London SW1X 8QG
0171 235 3325

Scotland:
21 Rutland Street
Edinburgh EH1 2AH
0131 229 3276
Provides home care and a day and night nursing service.

CEREBRAL PALSY
Scope
12 Park Crescent
London W1N 4EQ
0171 636 5020

CYSTIC FIBROSIS
Cystic Fibrosis Trust
Alexandra House
5 Blyth Road
Bromley
Kent BR1 3RS
0181 464 7211

DEAFNESS
RNID – Royal National Institute for Deaf People
19–23 Featherstone Street
London EC1Y 8SL
0171 296 8000/8001

DIABETES
British Diabetic Association
10 Queen Anne Street
London W1M 0BD
0171 323 1531

Scotland:
34 West George Street
4th floor
Glasgow G2 1DA
Tel: 0141 420 1759

DISABILITY
SPOD – Association to Aid the Sexual and Personal Relationships of People with a Disability
286 Camden Road
London N7 0BJ
0171 607 8851

Scotland:
Disability Scotland
5 Shandwick Place
Edinburgh EH2 4RG
0131 229 8632

Limbless Association
Roehampton Disability Centre
Roehampton Lane
London SW15 5PL
0181 788 1777

RADAR – Royal Association for Disability & Rehabilitation
12 City Forum
250 City Road
London EC1V 8AF
0171 250 3222

DOWN'S SYNDROME
Down's Syndrome Association
155 Mitcham Road
Tooting
London SW17 9PG
0181 682 4001

EPILEPSY

Epilepsy Association of Scotland
48 Govan Road
Glasgow G51 1JL
0141 427 4911

National Society for Epilepsy
Chalfont Centre for Epilepsy
Chalfont St Peter
Buckinghamshire SL9 0RJ
01494 601 300

HEART

British Heart Foundation
14 Fitzhardinge Street
London W1H 4DH
0171 935 0185

INCONTINENCE

Continence Foundation
2 Doughty Street
London WC1N 2PH
0171 404 6875
Helpline: 0191 213 0050
(*Mon–Fri 9.00–18.00*)

LARYNGECTOMY

Laryngectomy Association
Ground Floor
6 Rickett Street, Fulham
London SW6 1RU
Telephone and fax:
0171 381 9993

MENTAL HEALTH

MENCAP – The Royal Society for Mentally Handicapped Children and Adults
123 Golden Lane
London EC1Y 0RT
0171 454 0454

MIND – The National Association for Mental Health
15–19 Broadway
Stratford
London E15 4BQ
0181 519 2122

MOTOR NEURONE DISEASE

Motor Neurone Disease Association
PO Box 246
Northampton
NN1 2PR
01604 250 505
Helpline: 0345 626 262

MULTIPLE SCLEROSIS

Multiple Sclerosis Society of Great Britain and Northern Ireland
25 Effie Road
Fulham
London SW6 1EE
0171 610 7171

PARKINSON'S DISEASE

Parkinson's Disease Society of the UK
22 Upper Woburn Place
London WC1H 0RA
0171 383 3513

Scotland:
2 Claverhouse Drive
Edinburgh EH6 6BS
0131 477 3817

SCHIZOPHRENIA

National Schizophrenia Fellowship
28 Castle Street
Kingston Upon Thames
Surrey KT1 1SS
0181 547 3937
Advice line: 0181 974 6814
(*10.00–15.00*

SANE – Schizophrenia – A National Emergency
199–205 Old Marylebone Road
London NW1 5QP
0171 724 6520
London Helpline
0171 724 8000
(*14.00–24.00*)
Out of London Helpline
0345 678 000
(*14.00–24.00*)

SPEECH IMPAIRMENT

Royal College of Speech and Language Therapists
7 Bath Place
Rivington Street
London EC2A 3DR
0171 613 3855

STOMA

British Colostomy Association
15 Station Road
Reading RG1 1LG
0118 939 1537

STROKE

Chest, Heart, Stroke Association
63 North Castle Street
Edinburgh H2 3LT
0131 225 6963

The Stroke Association
Stroke House
Whitecross Street
London EC1Y 8JJ
0171 490 7999

ORGANISATIONS FOR THE ELDERLY

Action on Elder Abuse
Astral House
1268 London Road
London SW16 4ER
0181 679 2648
Helpline: 0181 679 7074

Age Concern
Astral House
1268 London Road
London SW16 4ER
0181 679 8000

Scotland:
113 Rose Street
Edinburgh EH2 3DT
0131 220 3345

Wales:
1 Cathedral Road
Cardiff CF1 9SD
01222 371 566

Help The Aged
16–18 St James Walk
London EC1R 0BE
0171 253 0253
Advice Line: 0800 650 065

SPECIALIST
EQUIPMENT

See also, **St. John Ambulance**
and **British Red Cross,** *who
loan equipment.*

Chester-Care and Homecraft
Sidings Road
Low Moor Estate
Kirkby in Ashfield
Notts NG17 7JZ
01623 757955
*Mail-order products for people who
are elderly, disabled or in pain.*

*Disabled Living Centres
Council*
1st Floor
Winchester House
11 Crammer Road
London SW9 6EJ
0171 820 0567
*Displays equipment for disabled
people, elderly people and carers.
They can tell you the location of
your nearest centre.*

Disabled Living Foundation
380–384 Harrow Road
London W9 2HU
0171 289 6111
Helpline: 0870 603 9177
Minicom: 0870 603 9176
*Information and advice about
equipment for disabilities.*

Keep Able
Freepost
Fleming Close, Park Farm
Wellingborough
Northants NN8 6BR
01933 679426
*Catalogue and advice line about
equipment for disabled people.*

COUNSELLING

*British Association For
Counselling*
1 Regent Place
Rugby
Warwickshire CV21 2PJ
01788 550 899
Provides a list of local counsellors.

*CRUSE – Bereavement
Care*
126 Sheen Road
Richmond
Surrey TW9 1UR
0181 940 4818
*Provides support and practical advice
for any bereaved person.*

Samaritans
10 The Grove
Slough, Bucks SL1 1QP
01753 532 713
For local branches:
0345 909 090
*Provides 24-hour helpline support to
anyone in distress.*

FINANCIAL AND
LEGAL ADVICE

Benefits Agency
Quarry House
Quarry Hill
Leeds LS2 7UA
0113 232 4000
Freephone Helpline:
0800 882 200

Benefits Enquiry Line
0800 882200

Court of Protection
Enquiries and Acceptance
Division
Public Trust Office
Protection Division
Stewart House
24 Kingsway
London WC2B 6JR
0171 269 7000
(See page 170)

Family Fund
PO Box 50
York YO1 2ZX
01904 621 115
*Provides financial help for families
with a severely disabled child.*

Health Service Ombudsman
11th Floor, Millbank Towers
Millbank
London SW1P 4QP
0171 217 4051

Scotland:
1st Floor
28 Thistle Street
Edinburgh EH2 1EN
0131 225 7465

Wales:
Pearl Assurance House
Greyfriars Road
Cardiff CF1 3AG
01222 394 621

The Law Society
50 Chancery Lane
London WC2A 1SX
0171 242 1222

*National Association of
Citizens Advice Bureaux –
CAB*
Myddleton House
115-123 Pentonville Road
London N1 9LZ
0171 833 2181

Scotland:
26 George Square
Edinburgh EH8 9LD
0131 667 0156

Patient's Association
8 Guilford Street
London WC1N 1DT
0171 242 1524

GLOSSARY OF MEDICAL CONDITIONS

Abscess A collection of pus anywhere in the body. A boil is a common type of abscess.

AIDS (Acquired Immune Deficiency Syndrome). A condition in which the immune system stops functioning properly. It is caused by infection with HIV (human immunodeficiency virus), which is transmitted sexually and through blood.

Alzheimer's disease A name given to forms of dementia (*see* Dementia) not resulting from disease of the brain's blood vessels. It results in loss of memory, confusion and unpredictable behaviour.

Anaemia A deficiency of haemoglobin, the red pigment in blood cells that carries oxygen around the body. The most usual cause is lack of iron. Symptoms include pallor and fatigue.

Angina Chest pain caused by narrowing of the blood vessels that supply the heart. When the demand for oxygen is increased, for example during exercise or stress, the affected heart does not receive enough oxygen, leading to pain.

Arthritis Inflammation of the joints. The joints, especially the protective cartilage and capsule, become diseased or worn out causing varying degrees of pain and disability. Two common types of arthritis are osteoarthritis and rheumatoid arthritis.

Asthma Attacks of wheezing and breathlessness which can become severe. It is caused by narrowing of the airways and is often triggered by an allergy, for example to pollen or to house dust.

Bronchitis Inflammation of the bronchi, the larger airways of the lungs. Common symptoms are breathlessness, coughing and production of phlegm. Acute bronchitis is usually short-lived and commonly follows a viral illness such as a cold, or inhalation of an irritant substance. Repeated attacks may result in chronic bronchitis, a permanent condition seen especially in smokers and those exposed repeatedly to air pollution.

Cancer A malignant tumour (growth) which, if untreated, can be fatal. Tumours can develop in any organ of the body, interfering with their function and destroying healthy tissue. Cells from the tumour can travel to other parts of the body to form secondary growths.

Cataract A disorder of the lens of the eye. The lens becomes opaque (milky in appearance), reducing the amount of light entering the eye. It may result in blindness.

Cerebral palsy Poor co-ordination and abnormal muscular control of various parts of the body due to brain damage, which most commonly takes place at birth.

Chickenpox An illness caused by the virus *herpes zoster*. Often described as a childhood illness, adults can also contract it. Symptoms include a high temperature, headache, and a red rash from which small blisters develop. The blisters are extremely irritating, but if they or their scabs are picked, permanent scarring can result.

Conjunctivitis Inflammation of the conjunctiva, the membrane that covers the front of the eye. It causes redness, itching and discharge from the eye.

Coronary thrombosis A blood clot in the arteries supplying the heart. It can occur suddenly, usually in arteries narrowed by disease. If the clot fails to dissolve quickly, part of the heart muscle dies, causing a heart attack (*myocardial infarction*). It is accompanied by severe central chest pain (*angina*) perhaps travelling to the neck and left arm, with profound shock and a feeling of doom.

Cystic fibrosis An inherited disorder that is usually present at birth. It affects various glands and is characterised by secretion of sticky mucus, repeated chest infections and failure to grow properly due to poor digestion of food.

Cystitis An acute inflammation of the bladder. Often caused by an infection, it causes lower abdominal pain together with painful and frequent passing of urine.

Dementia Gradual loss of intellect due to progressive deterioration of the brain cells. It is sometimes the result of deterioration of the brain's blood vessels and is usually, but not always, confined to the elderly. Dementia causes anxiety, memory loss and confusion.

Depression (depressive illness) An excessive down-swing of mood sometimes accompanied by lack of appetite, sleep disturbance and fatigue. Its seriousness is often under-estimated and medical advice should be sought.

Dermatitis Inflammation of the skin, a variety of which is known as eczema. It results in red, shiny, dry, cracked areas of skin. Scratching causes infection and weeping skin.

Diabetes A condition in which the pancreas secretes insufficient insulin or none at all. Symptoms include excessive thirst, frequent urination, weight loss, and in severe cases, it can lead to coma.

Eczema *See* Dermatitis.

Emphysema A disease of the lungs in which the small air sacs (*alveoli*) are destroyed. It causes breathlessness and can lead to heart failure. Often caused by smoking, emphysema also commonly accompanies chronic bronchitis and severe long-term asthma.

Epilepsy A condition in which periods of abnormal electrical activity in the brain can lead to seizures, loss of consciousness and possibly convulsions.

Gastroenteritis Inflammation of the stomach and bowel leading to diarrhoea and vomiting. It is normally due to a virus or eating contaminated food. Most cases will settle in 24 to 48 hours, but the condition can be more serious if the sufferer is very young or elderly, or if the symptoms are severe or prolonged.

Glandular fever A viral infection which characteristically results in swelling of the glands in the neck (*lymph nodes*). Other symptoms include high temperature and a sore throat.

Glaucoma A condition in which pressure builds up in the eyeball. It can lead to permanent damage and blindness.

Haemophilia A hereditary disease that affects males only, in which the blood fails to clot due to a lack of an ingredient known as Factor Eight.

Heart attack See Coronary thrombosis.

Hepatitis Inflammation of the liver caused by a viral infection. Hepatitis types A and E are transmitted mostly through drinking water contaminated by infected faeces. Hepatitis types B, C and D are transmitted through blood and sexual contact.

Herpes simplex A virus responsible for cold sores and genital herpes. It causes small blisters that erupt on the skin.

Herpes zoster *See* Chickenpox *and* Shingles.

Influenza (flu) An acute viral infection. Symptoms include high fever, sweating and muscle aches. In a healthy adult, the illness runs its course in seven to ten days and a full recovery usually results. Pneumonia is a dangerous complication, occurring more frequently in young children and the elderly.

Laryngitis Inflammation of the larynx (voice box). It results in a sore throat, cough and a hoarse or lost voice. Laryngitis is commonly associated with infections of the upper and lower respiratory tract but can also occur after misuse of the voice.

Leukaemia A cancer (*see* Cancer) that affects the white cells in the blood.

Measles A potentially dangerous viral illness, the characteristic symptoms of which are a rash and fever. It is more common in children.

Meningitis A bacterial or viral infection, that causes inflammation of the protective membranes (*meninges*) that surround the brain. Symptoms include severe headaches, avoidance of light, neck stiffness, nausea, vomiting, confusion and, in some cases, a reddish-purple rash. Bacterial meningitis can be severe and life-threatening.

Motor neurone disease A progressive disease affecting the nerves that control muscular activity. It usually appears in older people and results in increasing disability.

Multiple sclerosis A disease affecting the sheaths that protect particular nerves in the brain and spinal cord. It usually begins in early adulthood and progresses gradually with remissions. It causes weakness, poor co-ordination, loss of sensation and eye and bladder disturbances. Mood changes are common.

Mumps A viral illness occurring mainly in children. The characteristic symptom is painful swelling and inflammation of the salivary (*parotid*) glands, located just below the jaw.

Muscular dystrophy A group of hereditary disorders affecting the muscles (but not the nerves). They commonly affect children, causing progressive weakness and consequent deformities.

Osteoporosis A condition in which bone loses its density. When severe, it can cause bending and even fracture of the bones. Hormones have a strong influence on bone density and osteoporosis commonly occurs in women after the menopause because production of oestrogen has ceased.

Parkinson's disease A disease of the central nervous system. Due to lack of certain chemical substances in the brain, there is a progressive onset of muscular tremors and rigidity. Characteristic signs include trembling hands, slow speech and a stiff, shuffling walk. It usually occurs in the elderly.

Pneumonia An acute infection of the lungs. It is characterised by high fever, shivering and the production of infected green or yellow phlegm which may be blood-stained. The infection is usually caused by bacteria.

Polio A viral illness which, in a minority of cases, damages the motor nerves in the spinal cord causing paralysis of a limb or even of the muscles involved in breathing. Vaccination has now virtually eradicated the disease in many countries.

Rheumatism A commonly used term for joint and muscular aches and pains.

Scabies A skin infestation caused by a mite. It is spread by direct skin-to-skin contact. The mite burrows into the skin and causes an allergic reaction with intense irritation. Common sites affected are the finger-webs, wrists, elbows, armpits, the crutch and buttocks.

Shingles An illness caused by the virus *herpes zoster* which is also responsible for chickenpox. The virus affects nerves in the skin resulting in a painful, blistering rash. The sufferer remains infectious until the last blister has crusted over.

Sinusitis Inflammation of the sinuses (air-filled cavities around the nose). It is caused by an allergy or by an infection, and it may also follow a cold. Symptoms include pain behind the cheeks and the upper jaw. A build-up of fluid occurs which, if infected by bacteria, causes fever and the production of yellow-green mucus.

Spina bifida A defect present at birth in which one or more vertebrae has not developed completely and the spinal cord is exposed. It results in varying degrees of disability. Infection within the spinal canal is the most serious complication.

Stoma An opening in the body created surgically. If the voice box is removed, a stoma is created at the front of the neck through which the patient can breathe. Stomas are also made in the abdomen to collect faeces in patients with intestinal diseases.

Stroke Damage to the brain caused by a blood clot or haemorrhage. It can result in loss of consciousness or even coma, loss of speech and other bodily functions, and varying degrees of paralysis of different parts of the body.

Thrombosis A blood clot inside a blood vessel. If the thrombosis occurs in the brain, heart or lung, the person's life may be at risk. A clot forming in the leg may not be life-threatening in itself, but part of it may break off and travel to the lungs.

Tuberculosis (TB) An infectious, airborne disease that usually affects the lungs, causing coughing, chest pain and fever.

Whooping cough An infectious disease that mainly affects babies and young children, the main feature of which is distressing coughing fits and a cough that ends in a characteristic whooping noise.

INDEX

PERSONAL RECORD BOOK

USE THIS SECTION TO RECORD essential information about your relative's special needs, her likes and dislikes, and her daily and weekly routine. Once you have filled it in, it can be used by other people involved in your relative's care, such as volunteers or care professionals. It is designed to be used as a quick reference guide and should not replace a care plan (*see page 33*).

PERSONAL DETAILS

Full name

Date of birth

How he/she likes to be addressed

HOBBIES AND INTERESTS

Reading

Preferred newspaper/magazine/books

Television/radio

Preferred programmes

Other interests

COMMUNICATION NEEDS

Impaired speech

Details

Impaired sight

Details

Impaired hearing

Details

COMMUNICATION AIDS	
TYPE OF AID	WHERE IT IS KEPT

EMERGENCY INFORMATION

Relative/friend

Name

Address

☎

Neighbour

Name

Address

☎

Other carers

Name

☎

Name

☎

GP

Name

☎

District nurse

Name

☎

Other care professionals

Name

☎

Name

☎

Local hospital

Address

☎

EMERGENCY SERVICES
IN AN EMERGENCY DIAL 999

Address and directions to home

MEDICAL ESSENTIALS	
ITEM	WHERE IT IS KEPT
Medication	
First-aid kit	
Thermometer	

AROUND THE HOUSE

Gas

Mains shut-off

Water

Mains tap

Electricity

Fuse box

USEFUL TELEPHONE NUMBERS

Plumber

Name

☎

Electrician

Name

☎

Handyman

Name

☎

Gardener

Name

☎

Essential items

Spare keys are kept

Torch is kept

Candles are kept

Telephone

Telephones are situated

Heating

Central heating controls are

OTHER INFORMATION

EATING AND DRINKING

TYPICAL MEALS

Breakfast

Morning snacks

Lunch

Tea

Evening meal

Bedtime snacks

ASSISTANCE NEEDED

☐ None

☐ Uses aids

☐ Needs to be fed

Other information

DIETARY RESTRICTIONS

Health reasons

Allergies

Likes and dislikes

OTHER INFORMATION

EATING AND DRINKING AIDS

Fill in special cutlery or crockery used

TYPE OF AID	WHERE IT IS KEPT

PERSONAL CARE

WASHING AND BATHING

☐ No help needed

☐ Uses aids

☐ Needs assistance

Other information

DRESSING

☐ No help needed

☐ Uses aids

☐ Needs assistance

Other information

USING THE TOILET

☐ No help needed

☐ Uses aids

☐ Needs assistance

Other information

MOBILITY

☐ No help needed

☐ Uses aids

☐ Needs assistance

Other information

SPECIAL AIDS TO INCREASE INDEPENDENCE		
Give details of special aids that your relative uses or that help a carer to assist		
TASK	TYPE OF AID	WHERE IT IS KEPT
Washing and bathing		
Using the toilet		
Dressing		
Mobility		

DAILY ROUTINE

NOTE DOWN THE REGULAR TIMES that your relative carries out daily tasks, such as eats breakfast, gets dressed or just prefers to be left alone. Record any routines that a temporary carer should be aware of, so that the normal structure of the day is not affected if you are not there. Use the side panel to fill in details of the times that medication is required.

MORNING

....

....

AFTERNOON

....

....

EVENING

....

....

BEDTIME ROUTINE

....

....

MEDICATION TIMES

SPECIAL NOTES FOR NIGHT CARE

Fill in details, such as if your relative uses the toilet at night or needs to be turned in bed

....

....

....